BASED EMERGENCY ENT CARE

Second Edition

Andrew Lau

Thomas Jacques

Sankalap Tandon

Tristram Lesser

First published in the United Kingdom in 2007

Second edition published in 2015

Copyright © 2015 by Andrew S Lau, Thomas Jacques, Sankalap Tandon & Tristram H Lesser

All rights reserved

No part of this publication may be reproduced, stored in a retrieval system, or transmitted in any form or by any means, without the prior permission in writing of the publisher, nor be otherwise circulated in any form of binding or cover other than that in which it is published and without a similar condition including this condition being imposed on the subsequent purchaser.

ISBN: 978 1 5076 4597 0

ABOUT THE AUTHORS

Mr Andrew S Lau BSc (Hons), MB BS, MRCS (Eng), DOHNS is the Head and Neck Research Fellow at University Hospital Aintree and the University of Liverpool, United Kingdom (UK). He is also the creator and Editor of *entsho.com*.

Mr Thomas Jacques MB BS, MA (Cantab), MRCS (ENT) is a Specialty Registrar in Otorhinolaryngology, North Thames Rotation, UK. He is also Associate Editor of *entsho.com*.

Mr Sankalap Tandon BMedSci, BM BS, MD, FRCS (ORL-HNS) is a consultant head and neck surgeon at University Hospital Aintree, UK. He specialises in transoral laser microsurgery and thyroid surgery.

Mr Tristram H Lesser MS, FRCS is a consultant skull base surgeon at University Hospital Aintree, UK. He is a past Chair of the UK Otolaryngology Specialty Advisory Committee and convenor of the Merseyside ear surgery courses.

CONTENTS

Foreward   5

Introduction   7

Otology   11

Rhinology   41

Laryngology   63

Post-operative care   81

3

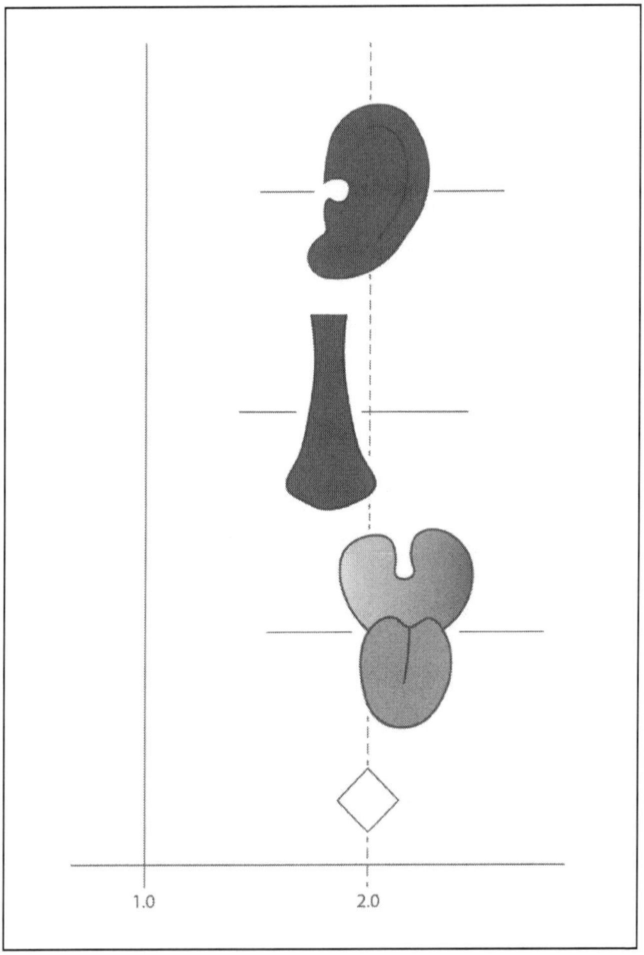
1.0
2.0

FOREWORD TO THE SECOND EDITION

The medical literature has changed significantly since the first edition was published eight years ago. In this time, a large number of new studies, Cochrane systematic reviews and National Institute for Health and Care Excellence (NICE) guidelines have been published or revised.

In light of this, we have revised and updated the text extensively. Where possible, we have used bullet points and have stratified our recommendations. Please refer to the Introduction (below) for a guide to our method and levels of recommendation.

We hope that this quick reference book will continue to aid colleagues, whatever their specialty.

ASL, March 2015

RELATED WEBSITE

http://entsho.com is a free educational website targeted at those working in primary care and emergency medicine and those cross-covering ENT. It provides an accessible, concise online reference, and is especially handy for out-of-hours work.

INTRODUCTION

Aim
This book is designed for use by practising clinicians involved in the management of ear, nose and throat (ENT) patients. It is aimed at 'first responders', by which we mean general practitioners, emergency nurse practitioners, emergency department doctors, ENT nurse practitioners and on-call doctors.

Our aim is to find and analyse published evidence for common ENT conditions and to provide management recommendations in summary form. While we would prefer to evaluate and analyse only high-quality evidence, frequently this does not exist in ENT. Consequently, we have taken a pragmatic approach and have also included moderate-quality evidence as well as common practice in the United Kingdom (UK).

We are aware that the medical literature is constantly changing and hope that this piece of work becomes a starting point for the individual clinician to remain up-to-date. We also hope that it stimulates readers to fill the evident shortfalls in many areas of ENT knowledge by undertaking their own high-quality research.

Evidence
Evidence was obtained from the Cochrane Library, the National Institute for Health and Care Excellence (NICE) website and the MEDLINE database through the PubMed search engine.

For analysis, papers were stratified according to the following levels of evidence:

I	Evidence from meta-analysis of randomised controlled trials, or from at least one randomised controlled trial.
II	Evidence from at least one controlled study without randomisation, or at least one other type of quasi-experimental study.
III	Evidence from non-experimental descriptive studies, such as comparative studies, correlation studies, and case control studies.

Evidence Levels IV and V amount to expert or consensus opinion.

Studies were assessed for the quality of research. Evidence was pooled where possible; studies of equivalent quality were included in discussion. Recommendations from Level IV and V sources were included as 'common practice'.

Recommendations

We were unable to consider cost effectiveness in making recommendations. Because of this, we have included relevant UK National Institute for Health and Care Excellence (NICE) guidance.

We decided to stratify our recommendations to reflect the quality of the evidence available:

Strongly recommended	Level I evidence for substantial net benefit
Recommended	Level I evidence for some net benefit
Suggested	Level II-III evidence for net benefit
Common practice	In widespread use and/or Level IV and V evidence for benefit
NICE Guidelines	NICE guidance including cost-effectiveness
Insufficient evidence	Insufficient evidence for or against use

Post-operative problems

Post-operative problems constitute a significant minority of emergency cases. Many patients with post-operative problems will present out-of-hours. We have included information on the expected post-operative course of a number of ENT procedures, as well as information on common complications.

As with much practical information, this section is not always directly evidence-based but represents non-controversial, typical UK-style management. These are general guidelines and we recommend that local (and individual consultant) policy for patient management should be sought wherever possible, including specific post-operative instructions from the operative note.

DISCLAIMER

This book is a reference resource intended for qualified and licensed doctors and nurses. The recommendations contained are the opinions of the authors. These are based on their own review of the medical literature and on current widespread medical practice in the UK.

Care has been taken to confirm that the information is, to the best of the authors' knowledge, accurate and up-to-date.

It is the practitioner's responsibility to determine appropriate clinical management with reference to senior or specialist colleagues, legislation, the medical literature and safety information. Practitioners should take into account the risks, benefits and side effects of treatments. Prescriptions and drug calculations should be checked with an authoritative source.

We strongly urge non-specialist practitioners to undergo formal training in general ENT. The authors, editors and publishers are not responsible for any errors, omissions or consequences arising from the use or misuse of the information in this publication.

OTOLOGY

ACUTE OTITIS EXTERNA (AOE)

Recommended
- Topical treatments alone are effective in uncomplicated AOE.[1]
    - Additional oral antibiotics are not required.
    - Antibiotic/steroid drops are more effective than placebo.
- Many antibiotic treatments seem to be equally effective and choice of topical treatment should be guided by side effect profile, risk of resistance etc.[1]
    - *eg* practitioners may choose to avoid gentamicin in those with a perforated tympanic membrane; refer to the British National Formulary (BNF).
- Instigate topical treatment for one week initially; continue treatment if symptoms persist, up to a maximum of two weeks.[1]
- Introduce alternate treatment if symptoms persist after two weeks' treatment.[1]

Suggested
- Stratify patients' risk of developing a complication and follow them up accordingly (see below); diabetic older men are at greater risk of complications.[2]
    - The vast majority (~95%) of AOE patients are managed in primary care.

Common practice
- The use of ear cleaning/microsuction is widespread in secondary care although there is little robust evidence for or against its use; the rationale is to clear debris to allow diagnosis and to improve penetration of antimicrobial therapy.
- In patients whose ear canals are occluded by inflammation, insertion of a (Pope or oto-) wick allows topical treatment to reach the canal; wicks are typically removed two to three days later.
- Some units advocate the use of glycerine-ichthammol-impregnated ribbon gauze; this mixture reduces canal wall oedema and has anti-Gram positive activity but does not provide significant anti-Pseudomonal cover.[3,4]
    - There is some evidence that clinic re-attendance rates are lower if using ribbon gauze packs.[5]
- If symptoms persist after two weeks' treatment, it is advisable to send a microbiological specimen for culture and to seek specialist help.

NICE Guidelines
- None.

ACUTE OTITIS EXTERNA (AOE)

Summary
Acute otitis externa (AOE) is a condition consisting of infection and inflammation of the external auditory canal (EAC). It is a common ENT problem constituting one in six new patient referrals, and 30% of follow-ups seen in one ENT emergency clinic.[6] Predisposing factors include loss of migration of epithelium of the EAC, change in the EAC pH and removal of wax production.[7] Swimming is another significant predisposing factor.[8,9] Infection is a major contributory factor to the condition, the commonest responsible organisms being *Pseudomonas aeruginosa*, *Staphylococcus aureus* and *S. epidermidis*.[8,10]

EAR Score
Evidence-based Acute otitis externa Referral Score

This scoring system seeks to highlight patients diagnosed with acute otitis externa (AOE) who are more likely to need specialist referral. It is not designed to take the place of a practitioner's clinical discretion or experience. Severely immune compromised patients eg those with neutropenia should be treated as per relevant guidelines.

1. Significant risk factors

One of	Age over 65 years	Score 1
	Recurrent AOE	
	Current chemo- or radiotherapy (not neutropenia – see above)	
	Diabetes mellitus (well controlled)	

Either	Immune compromise (eg HIV or transplant)	Score 2
Or	Diabetes mellitus (poorly controlled)	

2. Length of treatment

Either	Unplanned re-presentation with AOE symptoms in the first ten days of treatment	Score 3
Or	AOE not resolving for more than 14 days despite treatment	

3. Red flags

Please exclude the possibility of a primary neurological cause first

One of	Cranial nerve palsy	Score 5
	Disproportionate ipsilateral head pain	
	Erythema and swelling of the pinna or face	
	Completely stenosed ear canal (unable to insert speculum into ear canal at all)	

Key

Risk stratification	Total score	Recommendation
Lower risk	0	Unlikely to require specialist referral now. Patient can be discharged from initial consultation with prescription and safety-netting.
	1 – 2	Active monitoring appropriate. Patient progress should be reviewed in primary care during and after treatment.
	3 – 4	Consider a specialist referral for an emergency appointment within 12-48 hours.
	5+	Please make an urgent specialist referral.
Higher risk	Any red flag	

An audit and evidence-based guideline on the management of acute otitis externa in primary and secondary care.
Lau, Alexander, Medcalf, Khalil

ACUTE OTITIS EXTERNA (AOE)

References

1) Kaushik V, Malik T, Saeed SR. Interventions for acute otitis externa. *Cochrane Database Syst Rev.* 2010, Issue 1. Art. No.: CD004740. doi: 10.1002/14651858.CD004740.pub2.

2) Lau A, Alexander V, Medcalf M, Khalil H. An audit and evidence-based guideline on the management of acute otitis externa in primary and secondary care. Presented at ENT UK CAPAG Meeting 2010.

3) Nilssen E, Wormald PJ et al. Glycerol and ichthammol; medicinal solution or mythical potion? *J Laryngol Otol.* 1996 Apr;1 lO(4):319-21.

4) Ahmed K, Roberts ML et al. Antimicrobial activity of glycerine-ichthammol in otitis externa. *Clin Otolaryngol.* 1995 Jun;20(3)2201-03.

5) Pond F, McCarty D et al. Randomized trial on the treatment of oedematous acute otitis externa using ear wicks or ribbon gauze: clinical outcome and cost. *J Laryngol Otol.* 2002 Jun;116(6):415-19.

6) Raza SA, Denholm SW et al. An audit of the management of acute otitis externa in an ENT casualty clinic. *J Laryngol Otol.* 1995 Feb;109(2):130-33.

7) Jahn AF, Hawke Infections of the external ear. In: Otolaryngology-Head and Neck Surgery 2nd Edition. 1993 2787-2794. Mosby Year Book, St Louis, USA.

8) Agius AM, Pickles JM et al. A prospective study of otitis externa. *Clin Otolaryngol.*1992 Apr;17(2):150-54.

9) Springer GL, Shapiro ED. Fresh water swimming as a risk factor for otitis externa: a case—control study. *Arch Environ Health.* 1985 Jul-Aug;40(4):202-06.

10) Roland PS, Stroman DW. Microbiology of acute otitis externa. *Laryngoscope.* 2002 12(7 Pt 1):1166-77.

ACUTE OTITIS MEDIA (AOM)

Strongly recommended & NICE Guidelines
- NICE Clinical Guideline 69 (CG69)[1] makes use of a Cochrane Review meta-analysis[2] including thousands of patients.
- A 'no or delayed antibiotic prescribing strategy' should be used for the majority of those with AOM.
    - Over 80% of episodes of AOM resolve spontaneously and typical episode length is four days.
    - Compared to placebo, oral antibiotic therapy reduces pain at 2-7 days but number needed to benefit is high (20) and number needed to harm (vomiting, rash etc.) is lower (14).
    - When comparing oral antibiotic therapy with expectant observation, there were no significant differences between the outcomes for both groups.
    - Severe complications were rare and incidence was the same in both antibiotic-treated and placebo groups.
- Patients and parents should be counselled appropriately:
    - give advice on the length of an episode of AOM
    - give advice on prescription strategy
    - give safety net advice
- An 'immediate antibiotic prescribing strategy' should be used for those at high risk of complications including those:
    - systemically very unwell
    - with symptoms and signs of extra- and intra-cranial complications of AOM
    - with pre-existing co-morbidity such as significant cardiac disease, immune suppression and prematurity
- Depending on severity, an 'immediate antibiotic prescribing strategy' can also be considered for:
    - children with AOM and otorrhoea
    - children younger than two years with bilateral AOM.
- One Cochrane Review[3] found that shorter courses of antibiotics (less than seven days) had similar outcomes to longer courses.
- Prescribe pain relief and/or anti-pyretics

Recommended
- A Cochrane Review[4] found evidence that topical anaesthetic ear drops may benefit patients. Drug availability may be limited in the UK.
    - Pain 'diminishes rapidly' in any case with oral analgesics.

ACUTE OTITIS MEDIA (AOM)

Common practice
- Adults and adolescents with unilateral AOM should be followed up in clinic for otoscopy and nasendoscopy
- Patients with otorrhoea can be prescribed topical antibiotic drops

Summary
AOM is one of the commonest infections affecting humans. It occurs predominantly in younger children. Viruses are thought to be the usual causative organisms. The major complaint is of otalgia and management strategies are aimed at controlling this. Other common symptoms include (conductive) hearing loss, tinnitus, otorrhoea, malaise, anorexia and pyrexia.

Risk factors include male gender, age <7, bottle feeding, upper respiratory tract infection, immune suppression and craniofacial abnormalities. The condition is typically short-lived and self-limiting; a very small proportion of patients develop acute complications. Perforations of the tympanic membrane usually heal once the infection has been cleared.

Acute complications of AOM may be divided into extra- and intra-cranial types. Extra-cranial complications may include infections of the temporal bone (mastoiditis or petrositis), lower motor neuron facial palsy and rarely, abscesses of the neck muscles. Facial palsies usually occur in patients whose facial nerve canal bone is dehiscent as it passes through the middle ear. They resolve with corticosteroid treatment and treatment of the underlying AOM. Please see *Mastoiditis* below for more information.

Intra-cranial complications of AOM include meningitis, sigmoid sinus thrombosis and brain abscess. Note that otogenic brain infections may also occur in the absence of AOM or another acute ear pathology. In these cases, immediate ear surgery is not indicated.

ACUTE OTITIS MEDIA (AOM)

References

1) Respiratory tract infections – antibiotic prescribing. Clinical Guideline 69. National Institute for Health and Care Excellence. July 2008. Available from: https://www.nice.org.uk/guidance/cg69/resources/guidance-respiratory-tract-infections-antibiotic-prescribing-pdf. Accessed 1 October 2014.

2) Venekamp RP, Sanders S, Glasziou PP, Del Mar CB, Rovers MM. Antibiotics for acute otitis media in children. *Cochrane Database Syst Rev* 2013, Issue 1. Art. No.: CD000219. DOI: 10.1002/14651858.CD000219.pub3.

3) Kozyrskyj AL, Klassen TP, Moffatt M, Harvey K. Short-course antibiotics for acute otitis media. *Cochrane Database Syst Rev* 2010, Issue 9. Art. No.: CD001095. DOI: 10.1002/14651858.CD001095.pub2.

4) Foxlee R, Johansson AC, Wejfalk J, Dooley L, Del Mar CB. Topical analgesia for acute otitis media. *Cochrane Database Syst Rev* 2006, Issue 3. Art. No.: CD005657. DOI: 10.1002/14651858.CD005657.pub2.

AURICULAR HAEMATOMA

Suggested
- Auricular haematomata should be drained as early as possible (either by needle aspiration or incision and drainage), with application of a tight supportive head bandage and outpatient follow-up.[1-10]
- For recurrent haematomata, three case series[7-9] in a secondary care setting reported benefit from a bolsterless through-and-through mattress suture technique; 55 patients in total with one recurrence.
  - An older but tried-and-tested technique involves the use of cotton dental rolls, silastic splints and other bolster materials[4-6] to prevent further recurrence.
- One case series[10] set in an emergency department reports the use of an 18-gauge cannula for aspiration. The plastic component was left in place for several days before removal; the recurrence rate was three out of 53 patients; the main benefit is ease of use for non-specialists; there were no infections.

NICE Guidelines
- None.

Insufficient evidence
- Use of prophylactic antibiotics when the haematoma has been drained aseptically.
- A Cochrane systematic review[11] on interventions for acute auricular haematoma did not identify any randomised controlled trial, case controlled trials or cohort studies.

Summary
Auricular haematoma is a condition caused by collection of blood in the sub-perichondrial plane. It usually results from shearing trauma of the lateral surface of the auricle (also called the pinna). The posteromedial surface is less likely to develop a haematoma as there is a layer of loose areolar tissue under the skin. The presence of blood in the sub-perichondrial plane leads to interruption of the blood supply to the cartilage. This in turn predisposes to infection, chondronecrosis and the stimulation of mesenchymal cells, causing new cartilage formation. It is this that gives rise to the "cauliflower ear" deformity. This injury is seen most commonly in sports in which the player sustains forceful contact: rugby, wrestling and the like.

AURICULAR HAEMATOMA

References

1) Koopmann CF, Coulthard SW. Management of hematomas of the auricle. *Laryngoscope*. 1979;89:1172-4

2) Bull PD, Lancer JM. Treatment of auricular hematoma by suction drainage. *Clin Otolaryngol*. 1984;9: 355-360

3) Stark W, Kaltman S. Current concepts in the surgical management of traumatic auricular hematoma. *J Oral Maxillotac Surg*. 1992;50:800—802.

4) Henderson JM, Salama AR et al. Management of auricular hematoma using a thermoplastic splint. *Arch Oto Head Neck Surg*. 2000 July;126(7):888

5) Nahl SS, Kent SE et al. Treatment of auricular hematoma by silicone rubber splints. *J Laryngol Otol*. 1989;103:1146

6) Ho EC, Jajeh S, Molony N. Treatment of pinna haematoma with compression using Leonard buttons. *J Laryngol Otol*. 2007 June; 121(6): 595-6.

7) Roy S, Smith LP. A novel technique for treating auricular hematomas in mixed martial artists (ultimate fighters). *Am J Otolaryngol*. 2010 Jan-Feb; 31(1):21-4.

8) Kakarala K, Kieff DA. Bolsterless management for recurrent auricular hematomata. *Laryngoscope*. 2012 Jun; 122(6):1235-7.

9) Giles WC, Iverson KC, King JD, Hill FC, Woody EA, Bouknight AL. Incision and drainage followed by mattress suture repair of auricular hematoma. *Laryngoscope*. 2007 Dec; 117(12):2097-9.

10) Brickman K, Adams DZ, Akpunonu P, Adams SS, Zohn SF, Guinness M. Acute management of auricular hematoma: a novel approach and retrospective review. *Clin J Sport Med*. 2013 Jul; 23(4): 321-3.

11) Jones SEM, Mahendran S. Interventions for acute auricular haematoma. *Cochrane Database Syst Rev*. 2004, Issue 2. Updated 2011. doi:10.1002/14651858.CD004166.pub2

AURICULAR PERICHONDRITIS

Suggested
- Treat early with a broad spectrum systemic antibiotic with anti-Pseudomonal cover, *eg* ciprofloxacin.[1-3]
    - Beware the 1.6% risk of musculoskeletal adverse events with the use of systemic ciprofloxacin in the paediatric population.[4]

Common practice
- Depending on any associated signs of sepsis, oral antibiotic therapy with pain relief is adequate in many cases.
- If they are not hospitalised, it is prudent to follow-up patients until their perichondritis resolves; in one retrospective study[5], 7% of patients required debridement of necrotic tissue or abscess drainage.
- Drain auricular abscesses promptly as there is a high risk of subsequent cosmetic deformity ('cauliflower ear').
- Perichondritis can occur as a complication of otitis externa: treat the underlying cause (see *Acute Otitis Externa* above).

NICE Guidelines
- None.

Summary
Auricular perichondritis is an infective condition of the external ear. It is characterised by a painful, acutely inflamed and swollen auricle (pinna), which is exquisitely tender to touch. The commonest causative organism is *Pseudomonas aeruginosa*[1-3] although a minority of patients will have polymicrobial infections[5]. The condition arises as a result of trauma, as a sequel of otitis externa and after surgery of the external ear. Common traumatic factors include insect bites, trauma from hearing aid use and ear piercing, especially of the cartilaginous parts of the auricle (as opposed to the lobule).

AURICULAR PERICHONDRITIS

References

1) Martin R, Yonkers AJ, et al. Perichondritis of the ear. *Laryngoscope*. 1976;86:664-673.

2) Liu ZW, Chokkalingam P. Piercing associated perichondritis of the pinna: are we treating it correctly? *J Laryngol Otol*. 2013 May; 127(5):505-8.

3) Cumberworth VL, Hogarth TB. Hazards of ear-piercing procedures which traverse cartilage: a report of Pseudomonas perichoridritis and review of other complications. *BrJ Clin Pract*. 1990 Nov;44(11):512-3.

4) Adefurin A, Sammons H, Jacqz-Algrain E, Choonara I. Ciprofloxacin safety in paediatrics: a systematic review. *Arch Dis Child*. 2011 Sep; 96(6)874-80.

5) Davidi E, Paz A, Duchman H, Luntz M, Potasman I. Perichondritis of the auricle: analysis of 114 cases. *Isr Med Assoc J*. 2011 Jan;13(1):21-4.

BELL'S PALSY

Strongly recommended
- Bell's palsy patients should be treated with a combination of systemic corticosteroids (*eg* prednisolone 60mg daily, reducing over ten days) and anti-herpes antivirals (*eg* aciclovir 800mg five times daily for one week).[1-4]
    - A Cochrane systematic review[1] "shows that corticosteroids [alone] significantly increase the frequency of complete recovery" compared to control (n=1507, RR 0.71, 95% CI 0.61 to 0.83).
    - Patients receiving corticosteroids alone also had significant reduction in motor synkinesis.
    - A second Cochrane review[4] demonstrated significant benefit to patients receiving combined corticosteroid and antiviral treatment, when compared to placebo (n=658, RR 0.56, 95% CI 0.41 to 0.76).
    - Consider prescribing anti-acid prophylaxis when giving high-dose corticosteroid *eg* omeprazole.
- Do not prescribe antiviral therapy alone.[4]

Common practice
- It is important to prescribe artificial tears *eg* hypromellose and eye lubricant *eg* Lacrilube to those unable to close their eye; in addition, some practitioners provide eye shields and dressings tape.[2, 3]
    - If there are signs of corneal or other ocular trauma, consider referral to an ophthalmologist.
- Patients should be followed-up as outpatients two to three months after onset of Bell's palsy, with audiological assessment.

NICE Guidelines
- None.

Insufficient evidence
- Cochrane systematic reviews have found insufficient evidence for the utility of:
    - Acupuncture[5]
    - Acute surgical decompression of the facial nerve[6]
    - Physical therapy exercises and devices[7]
    - Hyperbaric oxygen therapy[8]

BELL'S PALSY

Summary
Bell's is a primary, idiopathic lower motor neuron facial palsy that is usually self-limiting. It is thought to be caused by inflammation of the seventh cranial nerve as it travels through the temporal bone. Some authors hypothesise that this is related to localised infection with herpes simplex virus. Clinically, Bell's palsy manifests as an isolated unilateral facial weakness of rapid onset, without forehead sparing. Associated features may include dry eyes, hyperacusis, motor synkinesis and an alteration in taste.[9] There are no other neurological features of a cerebrovascular event.

Bell's palsy has an overall incidence of 32 per 100,000 with a maximum incidence in the 15-45 age group. Spontaneous resolution of the weakness is seen in up to 71% of patients, with the majority of patients (58%) achieving this within 2 months.[10]

Note that facial nerve palsies secondary to trauma or infection are not Bell's palsies. Along with corticosteroids, treatment of the underlying cause typically leads to recovery.

BELL'S PALSY

References

1) Salinas RA, Alvarez G, Daly F, Ferreira J. Corticosteroids for Bell's palsy (idiopathic facial paralysis). *Cochrane Database Syst Rev*. 2010 Mar 17;(3)CD001942.

2) Gronseth GS, Paduga R; American Academy of Neurology. Evidence-based guideline update: steroids and antivirals for Bell palsy: report of the Guideline Development Subcommittee. *Neurology*. 2012 Nov; 79(22):2209-13.

3) Baugh RF, Basura RJ, Ishii LE Schwartz SR, Drumheller CM *et al*. American Academy of Otolaryngology clinical practice guideline: Bell's Palsy executive summary. *Otolaryngol Head Neck Surg*. 2013 Nov; 149(5):656-63.

4) Lockhart P, Daly F, Pitkethly M, Comerford N, Sullivan F. Antiviral treatment for Bell's palsy (idiopathic facial paralysis). *Cochrane Database Syst Rev*. 2009 Oct 7(4): CD001869.

5) Chen N, Zhou M, He L, Zhou D, Li N. Acupuncture for Bell's palsy. *Cochrane Database Syst Rev*. 2010 Aug 4(8):CD002914.

6) McAllister K, Walker D, Donnan PT, Swan I. Surgical interventions for the early management of Bell's palsy. *Cochrane Database Syst Rev*. 2013 Oct 16;10:CD007468.

7) Teixeira LJ, Valbuza JS, Prado GF. Physical therapy for Bell's palsy (idiopathic facial paralysis). *Cochrane Database Syst Rev*. 2001 Dec 7;(12):CD006283.

8) Holland NJ, Bernstein JM, Hamilton JW. Hyperbaric oxygen therapy for Bell's palsy. *Cochrane Database Syst Rev*. 2012 Feb 15;2:CD007288.

9) Rowlands S, Hooper R et al. The epidemiology and treatment of Bell's palsy in the UK. *Eur J Neurol* 2002;9(1):63-7.

10) Peitersen E. Bell's palsy: the spontaneous course of 2,500 peripheral facial nerve palsies of different etiologies. *Acta Otolaryngol* 2002;549 Suppl:4-30.

EXTERNAL AUDITORY CANAL FOREIGN BODY

Suggested
- Microscope-assisted extraction is preferable to direct vision.[1]
- Early referral to an experienced clinician or specialist service is advised
    - Inexperienced clinicians without specialist equipment have a higher failure rate[2]: in one case series[3], otolaryngologists had one-tenth the complication rate (lacerations, perforations etc.) of non-otolaryngologists.
- A technique using a cotton bud tip impregnated with tissue glue can be used for spherical object extraction[4] or dis-impacting the foreign body.[5]

Common practice
- Conventional wisdom is to drown live insects in surgical spirit; organic matter should not be wet given the risk of expansion and/or disintegration. Rigid foreign bodies can be flicked or hooked out.

NICE Guidelines
- None.

Insufficient evidence
- Use of prophylactic topical antibiotics following foreign body removal.

Summary
Aural foreign bodies are a common presentation. Foreign bodies vary from smooth objects such as beads or pebbles, through to organic matter such as insects and foodstuffs. Complications include ear canal injury and tympanic membrane perforation. Some evidence suggests that there is a correlation between handedness and the site of aural foreign body insertion *ie* right-handed children tend to present with foreign bodies in their right ear.[6]

EXTERNAL AUDITORY CANAL FOREIGN BODY

References

1) Schulze SL, Kerschnerl et a]. Pediatric external auditory canal foreign bodies: A review of 698 cases. Otol Head Neck Surg 2002;127(1):73-79.

2) Gregori D, Morra B, Berchialla P, Salerni L, Scarinzi C, Snidero S, Corradetti R, Passali D, ESFBI Study Group. Foreign bodies in the ears causing complications and requiring hospitalization in children 0-14 age: results from the ESFBI study. Auris Nasus Larynx. 2009 Feb;(36)1:7-14.

3) Olajide TG, Ologe FE, Arigbede OO. Management of foreign bodies in the ear: a retrospective review of 123 cases in Nigeria. Ear Nose Throat J. 2011 Nov;90(11):E16-9.

4) McLaughlin R, Ullah R et al. Comparative prospective study of foreign body removal from external auditory canals of cadavers with right angle hook or cyanoacrylate glue. Emerg Med J 2002;1 9(1):43-5.

5) Muzaffar SJ, Pollock JC, Sharp J. The troublesome aural foreign body – a useful technique. Clin Otolaryngol. 2011 Apr;36(2):186.

6) Peridis S, Athanasopoulos I, Salamoura M, Parpounas K, Koudoumnakis E, Economides J. Foreign bodies of the ear and nose in children and its correlation with right or left handed children. Int J Paediatr Otorhinolaryngol. 2009 Feb;73(2):205-8.

MASTOIDITIS

Common Practice
- In the UK, it is common practice to request urgent specialist assessment of patients who are likely to have mastoiditis.
- While they are being assessed, commence supportive treatment (intravenous fluids; analgesia; monitoring of vital and neurological signs).
- Start a broad-spectrum intravenous antibiotic to cover organisms such as *Streptococcus*, according to local policy.
- Keep the patient nil by mouth (NBM) in case there is an abscess that requires urgent surgical drainage.
- Consider a CT scan of the temporal bones to image both the middle ear/temporal bone and brain.
- Early involvement of other specialist teams (paediatrics, neurosurgery, radiology, anaesthetics) is very important.

NICE Guidelines
- None.

Summary
In the UK, mastoiditis is a *rare* but dangerous extra-cranial complication of otitis media. There is a recent history of otitis media and associated ear symptoms such as pain and discharge. The typical patient is septic; children are irritable, tug at the affected ear and stop feeding.

Symptoms indicative of mastoiditis include:
- Sepsis + severe otalgia + post-auricular swelling +/- ear discharge
- Cranial nerve palsy
- Altered neurological state *ie* drop in GCS or acute delirium

One of the justifications for prescribing antibiotics for acute otitis media is to prevent mastoiditis. A Cochrane Review[1] found that the incidence of severe complications in antibiotic-treated and placebo groups was the same. See *Acute Otitis Media* above.

MASTOIDITIS

References
1) Venekamp RP, Sanders S, Glasziou PP, Del Mar CB, Rovers MM. Antibiotics for acute otitis media in children. *Cochrane Database Syst Rev* 2013, Issue 1. Art. No.: CD000219. DOI: 10.1002/14651858.CD000219.pub3.

RAMSAY HUNT SYNDROME (RHS)

Suggested
- A short course of combination antiviral (*eg* aciclovir 800mg five times daily for one week) and corticosteroid therapy (*eg* prednisolone 60mg daily, reducing over ten days) probably improves outcome in Ramsay Hunt Syndrome (RHS).[1]
    - The evidence is somewhat mixed: the Cochrane Review on antivirals for RHS[2] only included one trial of low quality so could find no evidence of benefit.
    - The Cochrane Review on steroids for RHS[3] did not identify any trials suitable for analysis.
    - A different review by Dutch authors[1] included case series and cohort studies. It estimated that the recovery rate (House-Brackmann grade II or better) with combination treatment was 84% versus 38% without. There was, however, a higher risk of bias in the pooling of these data.
    - Consider prescribing anti-acid prophylaxis when giving high-dose corticosteroid *eg* omeprazole.
- Combination therapy should be started within three days of the onset of symptoms.

Common practice
- It is important to prescribe artificial tears *eg* hypromellose and eye lubricant *eg* Lacrilube to those unable to close their eye; in addition, some practitioners provide eye shields and dressings tape
    - If there are signs of corneal or other ocular trauma, consider referral to an ophthalmologist.
- Patients should be followed-up as outpatients two to three months after onset of RHS, with audiological assesment.

NICE Guidelines
- None.

RAMSAY HUNT SYNDROME (RHS)

Summary

Ramsay Hunt Syndrome (RHS; also known as herpes zoster oticus) is a condition caused by the varicella zoster virus. Reactivation of the virus in the geniculate ganglion causes a neuronitis and inflammation in the bony course of the facial nerve. This results in a unilateral facial palsy with the eruption of herpetic vesicles over the ipsilateral external ear, cheek or oral cavity. RHS may be associated with pain, hyperacusis, high frequency sensorineural hearing loss[4] and vertigo. [5, 6] It has an incidence of 2-5 per 100 000, with an increased incidence in the over-sixty age group and a slight female preponderance.

The severity of the facial nerve palsy is greater and the recovery profile is worse in RHS when compared with Bell's palsy.[3] In one series of RHS, complete paralysis was twice as frequent as incomplete paralysis and total recovery from complete and incomplete facial nerve palsy was 10% and 66% of patients respectively.[7]

Initial management includes oral medication as above and follow-up in clinic with audiological assessment.

RAMSAY HUNT SYNDROME (RHS)

References

1) De Ru JA, Van Benthem PPG. Combination therapy is preferable for patients with Ramsay Hunt Syndrome. *Otol Neurotol*. 2011; 32:852-5.

2) Uscategui T, Doree C, Chamberlain IJ, Burton MJ. Antiviral therapy for Ramsay Hunt syndrome (herpes zoster oticus with facial palsy) in adults. *Cochrane Database Sys Rev*. 2008, Issue 4. Art. No.: CD006851. DOI: 10.1002/14651858.CD006851.pub2.

3) Uscategui T, Doree C, Chamberlain IJ, Burton MJ. Corticosteroids as adjuvant to antiviral treatment in Ramsay Hunt syndrome (herpes zoster oticus with facial palsy) in adults. *Cochrane Database Sys Rev*. 2008, Issue 3. Art.No.: CD006852. DOI: 10.1002/14651858.CD006852.pub2.

4) Robillard RB, Hilsinger RL et al. Ramsay Hunt facial paralysis: clinical analyses of 185 patients. *Otolaryngol Head Neck Surg*.1986;95(1):292-297.

5) Kuhweiole R, Van de Steene V et a]. Ramsay Hunt syndrome: pathophysiology of cochleovestibular symptoms. *J Laryngol Otol*. 2002;116(10):844-8.

6) Adour KK. Otological complications of herpes zoster. *Ann Neurol*. 1994;35 Suppl 262-4.

7) Devriese PP, IVloesker WH. The natural history of facial paralysis in herpes zoster. *Clin Otolaryngol*.1988;13:289-298.

SUDDEN SENSORINEURAL HEARING LOSS (SSNHL)

Common practice
- It is common practice in the UK to prescribe a short course of oral steroids (*eg* prednisolone 60mg daily, reducing over ten days) for sudden sensorineural hearing loss (SSNHL).
    - Evidence is weak and studies are contradictory.
    - A Cochrane Review by Wei *et al*[1] included three trials with 'high risk of bias'. They had contradictory conclusions: two showed no effect while one showed significant improvement with oral steroid. There is therefore no review recommendation.
    - Moderate-quality (non-randomised but placebo-controlled) studies are also contradictory. Two[2,3] reported significant benefit from oral steroid while three[4-6] reported no benefit.
    - Consider prescribing anti-acid prophylaxis when giving high-dose corticosteroid *eg* omeprazole.
- Some randomised trials suggest that intratympanic steroid injection may benefit patients who have not responded to initial oral steroid.[7,8]
- There is no good evidence for the use of antivirals but this is common practice is some units.
    - A Cochrane Review[9] included four studies, none of which demonstrated any hearing improvement when different antivirals were used in addition to steroid.
- There is no good evidence for the use of vasodilators but this is common practice in some units.
    - A Cochrane Review[10] included trials with three different medications: results could not be combined. Individually, the three trials reported statistically significant benefit from carbogen, prostaglandin E1 and naftidrofuryl respectively, although patient numbers were small.
    - A number of lower-quality studies contradict these findings.

SUDDEN SENSORINEURAL HEARING LOSS (SSNHL)

Common practice (continued)
- There is some evidence for the use of hyperbaric oxygen therapy but access to such facilities is limited.
    - A Cochrane Review[11] included seven trials but could only pool data from two. There was a significantly increased chance of a 25% increase in the pure-tone audiometric average (RR 1.39; p = 0.02) though the 95% confidence interval was relatively broad (1.05 to 1.84). The number needed to treat was 5 with a confidence interval of 3 to 20.
    - Due to the low number of patients, the authors interpreted these results cautiously.
- Patients should undergo formal audiometric and otoscopic assessment at presentation and at follow-up appointments.
- Some patients may benefit from hearing aids and hearing therapy should their hearing not improve.

NICE Guidelines
- None.

Summary
SSNHL can be defined as a sensorineural hearing loss of 30 dB or more in at least three contiguous frequencies, developing within a three-day period.[2] It has an incidence of approximately 20 cases per 100,000 per year.[12] The peak age is in the 50-59 year group with a range of 10-79 and an equal sex distribution.[13] It is a condition of unknown aetiology with a number of theories as to its cause including vascular[14] or viral[15] events, and cochlear membrane breaks. A percentage of cases of sudden hearing loss are caused by acoustic neuroma, conductive hearing loss and syphilis. There is a high spontaneous resolution rate in this condition. Up to 65% of patients have a recovery to functional hearing without medical treatment.[13] The presence of vertigo may be a poor prognostic sign.

Management in the first instance is aimed at investigating identifiable causes for SSNHL and treating them as appropriate. Therapies in SSNHL are aimed at improving cochlear microcirculation and thus its oxygenation.

SUDDEN SENSORINEURAL HEARING LOSS (SSNHL)

References

1) Wei BPC, Stathopoulos D, O'Leary S. Steroids for idiopathic sudden sensorineural hearing loss. *Cochrane Database Syst Rev* 2013, Issue 7. Art. No.: CD003998. DOI: 10.1002/14651858.CD003998.pub3.

2) Wilson WR, Byl FM, Laird N. The efficacy of steroids in the treatment of idiopathic sudden hearing loss. A double-blind clinical study. *Arch Otolaryngol*. 1980 Dec;106(12):772-6.

3) Moskowitz D, Lee KJ, Smith HW. Steroid use in idiopathic sudden sensorineural hearing loss. *Laryngoscope*. 1984 May;94(5 Pt 1):664-6.

4) Kitajiri S1, Tabuchi K, Hiraumi H, Hirose T. Is corticosteroid therapy effective for sudden-onset sensorineural hearing loss at lower frequencies? *Arch Otolaryngol Head Neck Surg*. 2002 Apr;128(4):365-7.

5) Huang TS1, Chan ST, Ho TL, Su JL, Lee FP. Hypaque and steroids in the treatment of sudden sensorineural hearing loss. *Clin Otolaryngol Allied Sci*. 1989 Feb;14(1):45-51.

6) Edamatsu H, Hasegawa M, Oku T, Nigauri T, Kurita N, Watanabe I. Treatment of sudden deafness: carbon dioxide and oxygen inhalation and steroids. *Clin Otolaryngol Allied Sci*. 1985 Apr;10(2):69-72.

7) Wu HP, Chou YF, Yu SH, Wang CP, Hsu CJ, Chen PR. Intratympanic steroid injections as a salvage treatment for sudden sensorineural hearing loss: a randomized, double-blind, placebo-controlled study. *Otol Neurotol*. 2011 Jul;32(5):774-9. doi: 10.1097/MAO.0b013e31821fbdd1.

8) Plontke SK, Löwenheim H, Mertens J, Engel C, Meisner C, Weidner A, Zimmermann R, Preyer S, Koitschev A, Zenner HP. Randomized, double blind, placebo controlled trial on the safety and efficacy of continuous intratympanic dexamethasone delivered via a round window catheter for severe to profound sudden idiopathic sensorineural hearing loss after failure of systemic therapy. *Laryngoscope* 2009 Feb;119(2):359-69. doi: 10.1002/lary.20074.

9) Awad Z, Huins C, Pothier DD. Antivirals for idiopathic sudden sensorineural hearing loss. *Cochrane Database Syst Rev* 2012, Issue 8. Art. No.: CD006987. DOI: 10.1002/14651858.CD006987.pub2.

10) Agarwal L, Pothier DD. Vasodilators and vasoactive substances for idiopathic sudden sensorineural hearing loss. *Cochrane Database Syst Rev* 2009, Issue 4. Art. No.: CD003422. DOI: 10.1002/14651858.CD003422.pub4.

11) Bennett H, Kertesz T, Perleth M, Yeung P, Lehm JP. Hyperbaric oxygen for idiopathic sudden sensorineural hearing loss and tinnitus. *Cochrane Database Syst Rev* 2012, Issue 10. Art. No.: CD004739. DOI: 10.1002/14651858.CD004739.pub4.

SUDDEN SENSORINEURAL HEARING LOSS (SSNHL)

References (continued)

12) Byl JR. Sudden hearing loss: eight years" experience and suggested prognostic table. *Laryngoscope*. 1984 May;94(5):647-6i.

13) Mattox DE, Simmons FB. Natural history of sudden sensorineural hearing loss. *Ann Otol Rhinol Laryngol* 1977 Jul Aug;86(4 Pt 1):463-80.

14) Fisch U, Nagahara K et al. Sudden hearing loss: circulatory. *Am J Otol*. 1984 Oct;5(6):488-91.

15) Wilson WR, Veltri RW et al. Viral and epidemiologic studies of idiopathic sudden hearing ioss. *Otolaryngol Head Neck Surg*. 1983 Dec;91(6):653-8.

TRAUMATIC PERFORATION OF TYMPANIC MEMBRANE

Suggested
- Initially, active monitoring is appropriate given the high natural resolution rate. Patients with a perforation persisting for three months or more and a conductive hearing loss can be considered for surgical intervention.[1, 2]
  - One study[1] of 37 patients' non-blast-related perforations reported a spontaneous perforation closure rate of 88% within three months.
  - More recently, a study[2] of 114 patients revealed that 87% of blunt-force *and* blast-related perforations healed spontaneously within 12 months. The great majority (72%) of small- and medium-sized perforations had healed by the end of four weeks. A similar (70%) closure rate for larger perforations was achieved at eight weeks.

Common practice
- Perform an otoscopic examination and a pure tone audiogram to assess hearing loss and potential ossicular injury.
- If indicated by the mechanism of injury, assess and optimise the patient holistically according to Advanced Trauma Life Support principles.
  - A CT scan of the temporal bones/brain/spine may be warranted in major trauma.

NICE Guidelines
- None

Insufficient evidence
- Use of prophylactic antibiotics in otherwise uncomplicated perforations

TRAUMATIC PERFORATION OF TYMPANIC MEMBRANE

Summary
Tympanic membrane perforations commonly arise as a result of blunt force trauma applied over the external ear canal (*eg* road traffic collision or a slap to the side of the face). Perforations may also occur due to due to penetrating injury to the tympanic membrane. A third cause is barotrauma from scuba diving, explosions and forceful ear syringing.

Traumatic perforations occur commonly in a younger population with a female preponderance.[1] The resultant hole in the eardrum gives rise to symptoms of pain, hearing loss and serosanguinous discharge. Secondary infection may also occur.

Anecdotally, perforations tend to heal when dry – that is to say, when they are not infected. Consider using topical antibiotic drops if a pre-existing perforation becomes infected.

Perforations associated with chronic otitis media are not dealt with here.

References

1) Kristensen S, Juul A, Gammelgaard NP, Rasmussen OR. Traumatic tympanic membrane perforations: complications and management. *Ear Nose Throat J*. 1989 Jul;68(7):503-i6

2) Lou ZC, Tang YM, Yang J. A prospective study evaluating spontaneous healing of aetiology, size and type-different groups of traumatic tympanic membrane perforation. *Clin Otolaryngol*. 2011 Aug; 36:450-60.

RHINOLOGY

ACUTE RHINOSINUSITIS (ARS)

Strongly recommended
- *Uncomplicated ARS should be treated initially with symptomatic management only.* Antibiotic therapy has only modest clinical benefit, and is associated with significantly increased adverse events.
    - In a Cochrane review of nine RCTs, 86% of patients in the placebo arm experienced clinical cure or improvement, compared to 91% in the antibiotic arm.[1]
    - An earlier Cochrane review showed that antibiotics had a modest effect in shortening the duration of ARS compared to placebo (number needed to benefit = 18). There was a high rate of antibiotic-related adverse events (number needed to harm = 8), and a very low rate of sinusitis-related complications.[2]
- Paracetamol and/or NSAIDs should be recommended for symptomatic relief of discomfort and pyrexia in ARS.
    - An RCT showed significant improvements in headache, achiness and fever in participants receiving paracetamol or aspirin.[3]
- Antibiotics, if prescribed, should be of relatively narrow spectrum. A short (five to seven day) antibiotic course is likely to be as effective as a longer course of treatment, and may be associated with fewer adverse effects.
    - Co-amoxiclav may have a higher rate of adverse events.[1] A meta-analysis of RCTs found no difference between short (<7 days) and longer courses of antibiotics. The short-course group reported fewer side effects.[4,5]

Recommended
- Intranasal steroid sprays moderately improve symptoms of ARS, and may decrease the need for antibiotic treatment.
    - A systematic review of four RCTs examined the use of intranasal corticosteroids in ARS.[6] It concluded that there was a modest but statistically significant benefit of intranasal steroid administration in ARS.
- Systemic steroids have limited positive effects, but should be used cautiously in light of their potential side-effects.
    - A small clinical benefit of systemic steroid administration was found in a review of RCTs, with mild adverse effects.[7]

ACUTE RHINOSINUSITIS (ARS)

Recommended (continued)
- CT scanning is accurate, but should be reserved for complex cases where complications may be suspected.
    - A prospective cohort study showed that the diagnosis in ARS is made reliably by clinical assessment, and that CT contributes little to the management.[8]
- Plain radiographs are not useful in the management of ARS due to its poor specificity and sensitivity.
    - Plain radiographs have been shown in a prospective study to correlate poorly with CT images.[9]

Suggested
- Antibiotics may be considered in selected cases: patients with comorbidities or immune suppression, septic features, or if there are symptoms or signs suggesting bacterial infection: fever >38°C or severe (unilateral) facial pain.
    - Studies have suggested that high pyrexia and severe facial or dental pain are predictive of positive bacterial culture, although reports are contradictory.[10]
- Microbiology and other tests have limited usefulness in managing ARS.
    - The gold standard in diagnosis of ARS is sinus puncture and aspiration, although this is unnecessary in most settings. Raised serum inflammatory markers are associated with a higher rate of bacterial ARS, but their usefulness is unclear.[11] Nasendoscopy may not be available, but may help to identify purulent rhinorrhoea, which is associated with a higher rate of positive bacterial culture.

ACUTE RHINOSINUSITIS (ARS)

Insufficient evidence
- Nasal decongestant sprays provide symptomatic relief, but there is no evidence that they alter the disease course in ARS.
    - A controlled trial found that topical decongestant spray had no significant impact on the disease course in ARS.[12]
- There is little evidence of the efficacy of nasal saline irrigation in ARS.
    - A systematic review showed mixed results and highlighted the need for further studies.[13]

Summary
Acute rhinosinusitis (ARS) is subdivided into its viral form (the "common cold"), and its post-viral form, which may involve bacterial superinfection. ARS frequently arises from a viral upper respiratory tract infection. This causes mucosal oedema, which in turn causes blockage of the osteomeatal complex and stasis of mucosal secretions. Evidence-based management of ARS is reviewed comprehensively within the EPOS European Position Paper on Rhinosinusitis and Nasal Polyps 2012.[10]

ARS is defined symptomatically by the acute onset of symptoms including nasal blockage, rhinorrhoea, facial pain or pressure, and reduction in smell. Post-viral ARS is defined as the persistence of these symptoms beyond 10 days, or a worsening of symptoms after five days ("double sickening").

ACUTE RHINOSINUSITIS (ARS)

References

1) Ahovuo-Saloranta A, Rautakorpi UM et al. Antibiotics for acute maxillary sinusitis in adults. *Cochrane Database Syst Rev.* 2014 Feb 11;2:CD000243.

2) Lemiengre MB, van Driel ML et al. Antibiotics for clinically diagnosed acute rhinosinusitis in adults. *Cochrane Database Syst Rev.* 2012 Oct 17;10:CD006089.

3) Bachert C, Chuchalin AG et al. Aspirin compared with acetaminophen in the treatment of fever and other symptoms of upper respiratory tract infection in adults.... . *Clin Ther.* 2005 Jul;27(7):993-1003.

4) Gehanno P, Beauvillain C et al. Short therapy with amoxicillin-clavulanate and corticosteroids in acute sinusitis: results of a multicentre study in adults. *Scand J Infect Dis.* 2000;32(6):679-84.

5) Falagas ME, Karageorgopoulos DE et al. Effectiveness and safety of short vs. long duration of antibiotic therapy for acute bacterial sinusitis: a meta-analysis of randomized trials. *Br J Clin Pharmacol.* 2009 Feb;67(2):161-71.

6) Zalmanovici Trestioreanu A, Yaphe J. Intranasal steroids for acute sinusitis. *Cochrane Database Syst Rev.* 2013 Dec 2;12:CD005149.

7) Venekamp RP, Thompson MJ et al. Systemic corticosteroids for acute sinusitis. *Cochrane Database Syst Rev.* 2011 Dec 7;(12):CD008115.

8) Hansen JG, Lund E. The association between paranasal computerized tomography scans and symptoms and signs in a general practice population with acute maxillary sinusitis. *Apmis.* 2011 Jan;119(1):44-8.

9) McAlister WH, Lusk R et al. Comparison of plain radiographs and coronal CT scans in infants and children with recurrent sinusitis. *AJR Am J Roentgenol.* 1989 Dec;153(6):1259-64.

10) Fokkens WJ, Lund VJ et al. EPOS 2012: European position paper on rhinosinusitis and nasal polyps 2012. *Rhinol Suppl.* 2012 Mar;(23):3 1-298.

11) Hansen JG, Hojbjerg T et al. Symptoms and signs in culture-proven acute maxillary sinusitis in a general practice population. *Apmis.* 2009 Oct;117(10):724-9.

12) Inanli S, Ozturk O et al. The effects of topical agents of fluticasone propionate, oxymetazoline, and 3% and 0.9% sodium chloride solutions on mucociliary clearance in the therapy of acute bacterial rhinosinusitis in vivo. *Laryngoscope.* 2002;112(2):320- 5.

13) Kassel JC, King D et al. Saline nasal irrigation for acute upper respiratory tract infections. *Cochrane Database Syst Rev.* 2010 Mar 17;(3):CD006821.

EPISTAXIS

Strongly recommended
- Nasal packing with BIPP, tampon packs (e.g. Merocel) and pneumatic (Rapid Rhino) packs carry similar rates of cessation of bleeding.
    - There is no significant difference in effectiveness of bismuth iodoform paraffin paste (BIPP) impregnated ribbon gauze versus Merocel nasal tampons or inflatable packs in control of epistaxis.[1]
- Rapid Rhino packs are preferable to Merocel packs.
    - Three RCTs have compared inflatable nasal packs (Rapid Rhino) with non-inflatable nasal tampons.[2-4] They all showed that pneumatic packs are as effective as Merocel packs in stopping anterior epistaxis, but pain experienced on pack insertion and removal, and clinicians' ease of insertion and removal, were significantly better in Rapid Rhino pneumatic packs.
- Silver nitrate cautery and Naseptin are simple and effective first-line treatments for adult and child epistaxis, although their long-term efficacy is unclear.
    - An RCT found a significant decrease in bleeding in children treated with 4 weeks of Naseptin, compared with no treatment.[5] Naseptin cream and silver nitrate cautery show similar efficacy, whether used separately or in combination.[6,7] However, a retrospective cohort study showed that over of five years, recurrence rate of epistaxis is high, regardless of treatment.[8]
- Vaseline is not effective for paediatric epistaxis.
    - Petroleum jelly (Vaseline) used for four weeks conferred no benefit over observation, over an eight week period.[9]
- Tranexamic acid gel is not effective in epistaxis.
    - An RCT has shown treatment with tranexamic acid gel has no benefit over placebo at 30 minutes, 8 hours or 10 days after application.[10]

Recommended
- Endoscopic sphenopalatine artery (SPA) ligation is highly effective in controlling epistaxis which has not responded to nasal packing.
    - SPA ligation has been shown to be safe, and to have very high success rates immediately (93%), and at medium and long-term review, in two prospective observational trials.[11,12]

EPISTAXIS

Suggested
- Coagulation screen is not necessary unless there is anticoagulation, or persistent or recurrent bleeding.
  - Two observational studies have shown that, although a clotting screen is performed commonly in epistaxis patients, the result rarely alters the management if the patient is not on warfarin.[13,14]
- Warfarin therapy (unless out of control) or antiplatelet therapy should not be routinely stopped for patients admitted with epistaxis.
  - Srinivasan *et al.* [15] showed no significant increase in mean hospital stay in patients who continue on their warfarin therapy. The implementation of a guideline recommending the above management had no effect on re-bleeding or re-admission rates.[16]
- FloSeal® haemostatic matrix may have a role in decreasing the requirement for operative intervention.
  - The use of a human thrombin/gelatine matrix (FloSeal) has been shown to control epistaxis in 80% of patients who had failed to respond to nasal packing.[17]

Summary

Epistaxis (nosebleed) is one of the commonest emergencies seen by the otolaryngologist. It is a problem predominantly encountered at the extremes of age. Each group has different aetiologies and contributory factors. Anticoagulant (*eg* warfarin) and antiplatet (aspirin/clopidogrel) usage increase the risk of epistaxis, whereas use of other NSAIDs does not.[18] In the young, the bleeding tends to occur from the anterior septum secondary to nose-picking, resulting in crusting and local infection and inflammation. Bleeding in the adult population is usually idiopathic, due to a prominent vessel over Little's area giving rise to an anterior bleed; however, posterior bleeding can also occur.

Limited bleeding can be controlled with nasal cautery in the acute setting. Silver nitrate cautery is most often used in the treatment of recurrent epistaxis in the outpatient setting, along with topical antibiotic creams. In acute bleeding that does not settle with first-aid measures, nasal packing is the most commonly employed measure and is highly effective. In the event of further bleeding, operative management may be necessary; some new haemostatic products may represent an alternative to surgery in such cases.

EPISTAXIS

References

1) Corbridge RI, Djazaeri B et al. A prospective randomized controlled trial comparing the use of Merocel nasal tampons and BIPP in the control of acute epistaxis. *Clin Otolaryngol* 1995;20(4):305-7.

2) Badran K, Malik TH et al. Randomized controlled trial comparing Merocel and Rapid Rhino packing in the management of anterior epistaxis. *Clin Otolaryngol.* 2005 Aug;30(4):333-7.

3) Singer Al, Blanda M et al. Comparison of nasal tampons for the treatment of epistaxis in the emergency department: a randomized controlled trial. *Ann Emerg Med.* 2005 Feb;45(2):134-9.

4) Moumoulidis I, Draper MR, et al. A prospective randomised controlled trial comparing Merocel and Rapid Rhino nasal tampons in the treatment of epistaxis. *Eur Arch Otorhinolaryngol.* 2006 Aug;263(8):719-22.

5) Kubba H, MacAnolie C et al. A prospective, single-blind, randomized controlled trial of antiseptic cream for recurrent epistaxis in childhood. *Clin Otolaryngol* 2001;26(6):465-8.

6) Ozmen S, Ozmen OA. Is local ointment or cauterization more effective in childhood recurrent epistaxis. *Int J Pediatr Otorhinolaryngol.* 2012 Jun;76(6):783-6.

7) Murthy P, Niissen EL et al. A randomised clinical trial of antiseptic nasal carrier cream and silver nitrate cautery in the treatment of recurrent anterior epistaxis. *Clin Otolaryngol* 1999;24(3):228-31.

8) Robertson S, Kubba H. Long-term effectiveness of antiseptic cream for recurrent epistaxis in childhood: five-year follow up of a randomised, controlled trial. *J Laryngol Otol.* 2008 Oct;122(10):1084-7.

9) Loughran S, Spinou E et al. A prospective, single-blind, randomized controlled trial of petroleum jelly/Vaseline for recurrent paediatric epistaxis. *Clin Otolaryngol Allied Sci.* 2004 Jun;29(3):266-9.

10) Tibbelin A, Aust R et al. Effect of local tranexamic acid gel in the treatment of epistaxis. *ORLJ Otorhinolaryngol Relat Spec* 1995;57(4):207-9.

11) Abdelkader M, Leong SC et al. Endoscopic control of the sphenopalatine artery for epistaxis: long-term results. *J Laryngol Otol.* 2007 Aug;121(8):759-62.

12) Nouraei SA, Maani T et al. Outcome of endoscopic sphenopalatine artery occlusion for intractable epistaxis: a 10-year experience. *Laryngoscope.* 2007 Aug;117(8):1452-6.

13) Shakeel M, Trinidade A et al. Routine clotting screen has no role in the management of epistaxis: reiterating the point. *Eur Arch Otorhinolaryngol.* 2010 Oct;267(10):1641-4.

EPISTAXIS

References (continued)

14) Thaha MA, Niissen ELK *et al*. Routine coagulation screening in the management of emergency admission for epistaxis is it necessary? *J Laryngol Otol* 2000;114:38-40.

15) Srinivasan Patel H *et al*. Warfarin and epistaxis: should warfarin always be discontinued? *Clin Otolaryngol* 1997;22(6)2542-4.

16) Biggs TC, Baruah P *et al*. Treatment algorithm for oral anticoagulant and antiplatelet therapy in epistaxis patients. *J Laryngol Otol*. 2013 May;127(5):483-8.

17) Côté D, Barber B *et al*. FloSeal hemostatic matrix in persistent epistaxis: prospective clinical trial. *J Otolaryngol Head Neck Surg.* 2010 Jun;39(3):304-8.

18) Tay HL, Evans JM *et al*. Aspirin, non-steroidal anti-inflammatory drugs, and epistaxis. A regional record linkage case control study. *Ann Otol Rhinol Laryngol* 1998;107(8):671-4.

NASAL FOREIGN BODY

Recommended
- Positive pressure removal techniques should be tried in children in the first instance.
    - This is most commonly the "parent's kiss" technique. This method has a success rate of around 60%, with no adverse effects.[1] This technique may be less distressing, which allows further attempts with instruments in case of failure.[2]

Suggested
- Removal of posteriorly placed objects from the nasal cavity may be attempted with a Fogarty biliary balloon catheter.
    - A prospective trial showed 80% of patients had removal of the object on first attempt, with the remainder having a successful second attempt.[3]

Common practice
- Button batteries must be removed from the nose urgently.
    - Button batteries are a particular hazard if inserted into the nasal cavity. Effects vary from mild mucosal erosion, to nasal crusting, mucosal necrosis, rapid septal perforation and facial cellulitis.[4]

Summary
Nasal foreign bodies are a common paediatric otolaryngology referral; it is more common in children. It is most frequent in the two to six-year age range,[5-9] with some evidence for the right nostril being the choice for insertion (due to handedness).[7,8] The majority of patients present with a history of foreign body insertion. The remainder present later, commonly with a history of unilateral nasal discharge, which may be malodorous. Objects' location within the nasal cavity is usually along the floor or anterior to the middle turbinate. Occasionally, material may be found more posteriorly because attempts at removal have pushed it deeper into the nose.

NASAL FOREIGN BODY

References

1) Navitsky RC, Beamsley A et al. Nasal positive-pressure technique for nasal foreign body removal in children. *Am J Emerg Med.* 2002;20(2):103-4.

2) Botma M, Bader R et al. 'A parent's kiss': evaluating an unusual method for removing nasal foreign bodies in children. J Laryngol Otol. 2000;114(8):598-600.

3) Nandapalan V, McIlwain JC. Removal of nasal foreign bodies with a Fogarty biliary balloon catheter. *J Laryngol Otol.* 1994;108(9):758-60.

4) Loh WS, Leong JL et al. Hazardous foreign bodies: complications and management of button batteries in nose. *Ann Otol Rhinol Laryngol.* 2003;112(4):379-83

5) Baker MD. Foreign bodies of the ears and nose in childhood. *Pediatr Emerg Care.* 1987;3(2):67-70.

6) Tong MCF, Ying SY et al. Nasal foreign bodies in children. *Int J Pediatr Otorhinolaryngol.* 1996;35(3):207-11.

7) Francois M, Harnrioui R et al. Nasal foreign bodies in children. *Eur Arch Otorhinolaryngol.* 1998;255(3):132-4.

8) Hon SK, Izarn TM et al. A prospective evaluation of foreign bodies presenting to the Ear, Nose and Throat Clinic, Hospital Kuala Lumpur. *Medi Malaysia.* 2001;56(4):463—70.

9) Persaud R, Narula A et al. Foreign bodies. *BMJ.* 2014 Jan 30;348:g391.

NASAL FRACTURE

Strongly recommended
- Closed manipulation under anaesthesia may be performed under general or local anaesthesia, with comparable outcomes.
    - An RCT comparing local *vs* general anaesthesia showed no significant difference in perioperative pain scores or the need for subsequent septorhinoplasty between the two groups.[1]
- Local anaesthesia can be delivered topically or by infiltration; topical administration is slower, but may be less painful overall.
    - An RCT shows a significant decrease in pain experienced by patients having topical local anaesthetic compared with infiltration. The topical anaesthesia group required a minimum of 20 minutes for anaesthesia to be effective.[2]

Suggested
- Open reduction of nasal fractures is effective, and may be suited to the management of more severe deformities.
    - A retrospective study of 86 patients found that open reduction is more often performed for severe deformities, with similar success rates (as defined by the need for revision surgery).[3]
- Patients can be allowed to assess nasal deviation themselves and self-refer if desired, as long as sufficient flexibility is available to compensate for any delay this may create.
    - Patients should be advised in A&E of the local ENT protocol. Patients' own assessment of acquired nasal deviations is as accurate as those of clinicians. It is therefore likely to be safe to given patients contact information to allow self-referral in the period after injury.[4] There was no difference in airway or cosmetic outcomes, despite the potential for increased delay.
- Delays to manipulation should be minimised as this increases the rate of success. It is common practice to review a patient 5-7 days after injury.
    - Earlier intervention with manipulation under anaesthesia has been shown to be associated with higher patient satisfaction, in a prospective observational study.[5]
- Clinic assessment can be reliably carried out by junior doctors or experienced nurse practitioners.[6]

NASAL FRACTURE

Summary

Nasal fractures are a common part of the day-to-day ENT workload. They are commonest among the young male population, and are a clinical diagnosis. The fracture may be undisplaced, depressed or displaced laterally. Treatment is dependent on the patient's wishes and on alteration in appearance.

Management options include no treatment, closed reduction or open reduction. These may be done under local or general anaesthetic. Common practice in the UK is to perform closed reduction under local or general anaesthesia, within 2-3 weeks of injury.

NASAL FRACTURE

References

1) Khwaja S, Pahade AV *et al*. Nasal fracture reduction: local versus general anaesthesia. *Rhinology.* 2007;45(1):83-8.

2) Jones TM, Nandapalan V. Manipulation of the fractured nose: a comparison of local infiltration anaesthesia and topical local anaesthesia. *Clin Otolaryngol.* 1999;24(5):443-6.

3) Ondik MP, Lipinski L *et al*. The treatment of nasal fractures: a changing paradigm. *Arch Facial Plast Surg.* 2009;11(5):296-302.

4) Baring DE, Bowyer DJ *et al*. Patient self-assessment of nasal fractures and self-referral to an ear, nose, and throat department: a prospective study. *Otolaryngol Head Neck Surg.* 2012;146(6):913-7.

5) Yilmaz MS, Guven M *et al*. Nasal fractures: is closed reduction satisfying? *J Craniofac Surg.* 2013;24(1):36-8.

6) Baring D, Murray C *et al*. Prospective, blinded study of nasal injuries: comparison of doctor and nurse assessment. *J Laryngol Otol.* 2009;123(12):1338-42.

PERIORBITAL CELLULITIS

Recommended
Evidence in orbital cellulitis is limited by the seriousness of the condition.
- Blood cultures and nasal cavity or conjunctival swabs are of limited use.
    - Only abscess cavity swabs give significant yield; other swabs may be positive but often represent normal flora.[1-5]
- Lumbar puncture should not routinely be undertaken unless central neurological signs are present (after exclusion of raised intracranial pressure).[3,5]

Suggested
- History and examination are the mainstay of diagnosis of orbital infections. The key distinction is whether there is involvement of the area posterior to the orbital septum.
    - Post-septal infection is commonly due to sinus infection, whereas pre-septal infection is most often due to local skin trauma such as insect bites or dacrocystitis [6].
    - The clinical signs of post-septal infection include chemosis, ophthalmoplegia, painful extra-ocular movements, proptosis, loss of red colour vision and reduction in visual acuity. Ophthalmoplegia and proptosis have a positive predictive value for of 97% and a negative predictive value of 93% [7].
- Patients with signs of post-septal infection, especially ophthalmoplegia and proptosis, should undergo urgent CT scanning to exclude extraconal or intraconal abscess, intracranial or cavernous sinus involvement.
    - Two retrospective studies[8,9] found that CT correctly identified the final surgical diagnosis in 84% of patients. If a patient fails to improve or deteriorates despite CT findings of no collection, then re-scanning or surgical intervention is warranted.
- Proven subperiosteal or orbital collections should be drained urgently via an endoscopic or open approach, dependent on the surgeon's safest practice.
    - Surgical drainage of a collection may be undertaken via a Lynch-Howarth incision, or via an endoscopic approach.[10-13] Superiorly-sited collections may more often be treated via the external route, whilst medially-placed abscesses are often tackled endoscopically.[10,12]
- Small (< 10mm) medial subperiosteal collections, without significant adverse eye signs, may respond to intravenous antibiotic treatment – however this requires highly vigilant care.

PERIORBITAL CELLULITIS

Suggested (continued)
- A systematic review showed that 57% of patients with post-septal disease were managed successfully without surgical intervention. These patients, however, require very close ENT and ophthalmology monitoring to allow rapid surgical intervention.[6]

Common practice
- Antibiotic therapy should be commenced urgently, covering the commonest causative bacteria i.e. a third-generation cephalosporin and metronidazole.
  - The commonest organisms isolated are staphylococcal and streptococcal species and mixed anaerobes.[1,2,5,14-15] *Haemophilus influenzae* type B (HiB) is now uncommon due to vaccination.[4]

PERIORBITAL CELLULITIS

Summary
Periorbital and orbital cellulitis are acute infective conditions of the eyelid and the contents of the orbit, respectively. They may arise as a result of spread of infection from structures adjacent to the eye due to skin trauma, acute dacryocystitis, chalazion, facial cellulitis or severe infective conjunctivitis, or may occur as a complication of acute or chronic rhinosinusitis. Orbital infection is the most common complication of rhinosinusitis.

The management of orbital complications of acute rhinosinusitis is reviewed comprehensively in the EPOS European Position Paper on Rhinosinusitis and Nasal Polyps 2012.[16]

The Chandler classification of orbital complications of rhinosinusitis is frequently cited in discussion of periorbital and orbital infections, and has five grades:[17]

Grade I	Preseptal cellulitis
Grade II	Orbital cellulitis
Grade III	Subperiosteal abscess
Grade IV	Orbital abscess
Grade V	Cavernous sinus thrombosis/ central nervous system complications

The Chandler classification should be viewed as *categories* of periorbital infection, *not* as a pattern of disease progression. Preseptal cellulitis often has a different aetiology to orbital infections, and rarely progresses directly to the other stages. Likewise, cavernous sinus thrombosis is more often associated with sphenoiditis than frontal or ethmoidal infection, and may represent a distinct condition.[18]

The priority in management of orbital complications of rhinosinusitis is to distinguish promptly between preseptal cellulitis, which does not threaten the eye, and can be managed with intravenous antibiotics, and postseptal (orbital) infection, which may require emergency surgery to prevent visual loss.

The absence of any of these signs suggests pre-septal infection – the patient may be managed initially with IV antibiotics with close clinical review. The presence of any adverse eye signs, inability to assess the eye fully, or failure to improve after 24 hours of intravenous antibiotics, should prompt urgent imaging.

PERIORBITAL CELLULITIS

References

1) Ferguson MP, McNab AA. Current treatment and outcome in orbital cellulitis. *Aust N Z Ophthalmol.* 1999 Dec;27(6):375-9.

2) Schramm VL Jr, Curtin HD et al. Evaluation of orbital cellulitis and results of treatment. *Laryngoscope.* 1982(7 Pt 1):732-8.

3) Schwartz GR, Wright SW. Changing bacteriology of periorbital cellulitis. *Ann Emerg Med.* 1996 Dec;28(6):617-20.

4) Ambati BK, Ambati J et al. Periorbital and orbital cellulitis before and after the advent of Haemophilus influenzae type B vaccination. *Ophthalmology.* 2000 Aug;107(8):1450-3.

5) Uzcategui N, Warman R et al. Clinical practice guidelines for the management of orbital cellulitis. *J Pediatr Ophthalmol Strabismus.* 1998 Mar-Apr;35(2):73-9.

6) Baring DE, Hilmi OJ. An evidence based review of periorbital cellulitis. *Clin Otolaryngol.* 2011 Feb;36(1):57-64.

7) Soboi SE, Marchand J et al. Orbital complications of sinusitis in children. *J Otolaryngol.* 2002 Jun;31(3):131-6.

8) Clary RA, Cunningham MJ et al. Orbital complications of acute sinusitis: comparison of computed tomography scan and surgical findings. *Ann Otol Rhinol Laryngol.* 1992 Jul;101(7):598-600.

9) Patt BS, Manning SC. Blindness resulting from orbital complications of sinusitis. *Otolaryngol Head Neck Surg.* 1991 Jun;104(6)3789-95.

10) Rahbar R, Robson CD et al. Management of orbital subperiosteal abscess in children. *Arch Otolaryngol Head Neck Surg.* 2001 Mar;127(3):281-6.

11) Page EL, Wiatrak BJ. Endoscopic vs external drainage of orbital subperiosteal abscess. *Arch Otolaryngol Head Neck Surg.* 1996 Jul;122(7):737-40.

12) Ikeda K, Oshima T et al. Surgical treatment of subperiosteal abscess of the orbit: Sendai's ten-year experience. *Auris Nasus Larynx.* 2003 Aug;30(3):259-62.

13) Noordzij JP, Harrison SE et al. Pitfalls in the endoscopic drainage of subperiosteal orbital abscesses secondary to sinusitis. *Am J Rhinol.* 2002 Mar-Apr;16(2):97-101.

14) Donahue SP, Schwartz G. Preseptal and orbital cellulitis in childhood. A changing microbiologic spectrum. *Ophthalmology.* 1998 Oct;105(10):1902-5.

15) Kanra G, Secmeer G et al. Periorbital cellulitis: a comparison of different treatment regimens. *Acta Paediatr Jpn.* 1996 Aug;38(4):339-42.

PERIORBITAL CELLULITIS

References (continued)

16) Fokkens WJ, Lund VJ et al. EPOS 2012: European position paper on rhinosinusitis and nasal polyps 2012. *Rhinol Suppl.* 2012 Mar;(23):3 1-298.

17) Chandler JR, Langenbrunner DJ et al. The pathogenesis of orbital complications in acute sinusitis. Laryngoscope. 1970 Sep;80(9):1414-28.

18) Osborn MK, Steinberg JP. Subdural empyema and other suppurative complications of paranasal sinusitis. Lancet Infect Dis. 2007 Jan;7(1):62-7.

SEPTAL HAEMATOMA AND ABSCESS

Suggested
- Septal haematoma or abscess can be drained under either local or general anaesthesia.[1-3]

Common practice
- Septal haematomas and abscesses should be drained.
    - Haematomas and abscesses deprive the septal cartilage of its blood supply, which may lead to septal perforation or saddle deformity.
    - Reports describe a variety of drainage systems including Penrose drain insertion[1,2] and suction drainage.[4]
- Septal abscess should be co-treated with antibiotics.
    - Established abscesses are generally treated with intravenous antibiotics at the outset. The common organisms cultured from abscesses are *S. aureus*, *S. pneumoniae* and group A *Streptococcus*.[2, 5, 6]
- In septal haematoma, prophylactic antibiotic cover for staphylococcal and streptococcal species is frequently given, although no evidence for this exists.

Summary
Septal haematoma is a collection of blood in the sub-mucoperichondrial plane. The haematoma elevates the perichondrium off the cartilage and increases the pressure in this plane. Haematomas are typically caused by trauma or septal surgery. Abscesses may occur from secondary infection of an established haematoma, or *de novo* from infections such as vestibulitis[6] or furunculosis[1]. Both conditions are typically treated with open drainage, with approximation of the septal flaps to prevent re-accumulation.

SEPTAL HAEMATOMA AND ABSCESS

References

1) Arnbrus PS, Eavey RD et al. Management of nasal septal abscess. *Laryngoscope*. 1981;91(4):575-82.

2) Alvarez H, Osorio J et al. Sequelae after nasal septum injuries in children. *Auris Nasus Larynx*. 2000;27(4):339-42.

3) Kryger H, Dommerby H. Haematoma and abscess of the nasal septum. *Clin Otolaryngol*. 1987;12(2):125-9.

4) Carraway JH, Mellow CG. Simple suction drainage: an adjunct to septal surgery. *Ann Plast Surg*. 1990;24(2):191-3.

5) Canty PA, Berkowitz RG. Hematoma and abscess of the nasal septum in children. *Arch Otolaryngol Head Neck Surg*. 1996;122(12):1373-6.

6) Jalaludin MA. Nasal septal abscess – retrospective analysis of 14 cases from University Hospital, Kuala Lumpur. *Singapore Med J*. 1993;34(5):435-7.

LARYNGOLOGY

ACUTE TONSILLITIS AND SORE THROAT

Primary Care & Emergency Medicine:
Strongly Recommended & NICE Guidelines
- NICE Clinical Guideline 69 (CG69)[1] addresses the use of antibiotics in sore throat.
- A 'no or delayed antibiotic prescribing strategy' should be used for the majority of those with acute tonsillitis, sore throat or pharyngitis.
    - Many episodes of sore throat are viral in origin and typical episode length is one week.
- Patients and parents should be counselled appropriately:
    - give advice on the length of an episode of sore throat
    - give advice on prescription strategy
    - give safety net advice
- An 'immediate antibiotic prescribing strategy' should be used for those at high risk of complications including those:
    - systemically very unwell
    - with symptoms and signs of peritonsillar abscess, epiglottitis or deep neck space abscess
    - with pre-existing co-morbidity such as significant cardiac disease, immune suppression and prematurity
- An 'immediate antibiotic prescribing strategy' can also be considered for patients exhibiting three or more Centor criteria.
- Modified Centor criteria can be used to determine the likelihood of a bacterial aetiology in adults[2] (but not in children[3]):
    - Online resource: http://www.mdcalc.com/modified-centor-score-for-strep-pharyngitis/
- In those likely to have Group A streptoccocal tonsillopharyngitis:
    - Pencillins should be considered first choice (unless allergic). One Cochrane Review[4] concluded that they have a similar clinical efficacy to cephalosporins and macrolides; macrolides are associated with more adverse events.
    - Shorter courses of antibiotics can be used. One Cochrane Review[5] concluded that three- to six-day courses of antibiotics have comparable clinically efficacy to ten-day courses. Both groups had a similar risk (of the order of 0.01%) of developing a late complication (*eg* glomerulonephritis).

ACUTE TONSILLITIS AND SORE THROAT

Primary Care & Emergency Medicine:
Strongly Recommended & NICE Guidelines (continued)
- Prescribe a single dose of corticosteroid as an adjunct to any antibiotics. A Cochrane Review[6] found that add-on steroid greatly increased the likelihood of complete resolution of pain at 24 hours (RR 3.2; 95% CI 2 to 5.1; p<0.001; number needed to benefit <4).
  - The majority of trials studied used a single dose of 60mg prednisolone or 10mg dexamethasone.
  - Trials did not include patients with peritonsillar abscess and infectious mononucleosis
- For recurrent acute sore throats: counsel patients according to SIGN Guideline 117.[7]

Secondary Care: Common Practice
- Admit patients who cannot swallow sips of fluids regularly (including antibiotic or analgesic suspension).
- Establish a clinical diagnosis and request a glandular fever screen and full blood count; routine throat swabs are not indicated.
- Fluid resuscitate the patient: young, fit, dehydrated patients seem to benefit from active intravenous rehydration.
- Prescribe intravenous antibiotics according to local policy; common regimes include: IV benzylpenicillin 1.2g qds with metronidazole 500mg tds *or* IV clarithromycin 500mg bd if pencillin allergic.
- Switch to oral antibiotic and analgesic therapy as soon as swallowing improves; actively encourage a return to normal diet including more fibrous solids like toast and porridge (rather than ice cream).

Summary
Most sore throats are viral but it can be difficult to make a distinction between viral and bacterial tonsillopharyngitis clinically. Acute tonsillitis is an infection of the palatine tonsils. It occurs alone, or as part of a wider tonsillopharyngitis. Diagnosis is based on a history of pyrexia, sore throat, odynophagia and dysphagia. Examination reveals acutely inflamed tonsils with exudate, which may also be associated with inflammation of the pharynx. Tender cervical lymphadenopathy may be present.

Treatment is aimed at symptom control. Antibiotic therapy may be indicated in resistant cases or where the patient is at high risk of complications. Common causative bacteria include Group A beta-haemolytic *Streptococci* (GABHS). The widespread use of antibiotics has probably led to the misperception that sore throats are all bacterial in origin.

ACUTE TONSILLITIS AND SORE THROAT

References

1) Respiratory tract infections – antibiotic prescribing. Clinical Guideline 69. National Institute for Health and Care Excellence. July 2008. Available from: https://www.nice.org.uk/guidance/cg69/resources/guidance-respiratory-tract-infections-antibiotic-prescribing-pdf. Accessed 1 October 2014.

2) Centor RM, Witherspoon JM, Dalton HP, Brody CE & Link K. The diagnosis of strep throat in adults in the emergency room. *Med Decision Making*. 1981. **1** (3): 239–246. doi:10.1177/0272989x8100100304.

3) Roggen I, van Berlaer G, Gordts F, Hubloue I. Centor Criteria, For what it's worth. *BMJ Open*. 2013. **3** (4): e002712. doi:10.1136/bmjopen-2013-002712.

4) vanDriel ML, De Sutter AIM, Keber N, Habraken H, Christiaens T. Different antibiotic treatments for group A streptococcal pharyngitis. *Cochrane Database Syst Rev*. 2013, Issue 4. Art. No.: CD004406. DOI: 10.1002/14651858.CD004406.pub3.

5) Altamimi S, Khalil A, Khalaiwi KA, Milner RA, Pusic MV, Al Othman MA. Short-term late-generation antibiotics versus longer term penicillin for acute streptococcal pharyngitis in children. *Cochrane Database of Syst Rev*. 2012. Issue 8. Art. No.: CD004872. DOI: 10.1002/14651858.CD004872.pub3.

6) Hayward G, Thompson MJ, Perera R, Glasziou PP, Del Mar CB, Heneghan CJ. Corticosteroids as standalone or add-on treatment for sore throat. *Cochrane Database of Syst Rev*. 2012. Issue 10. Art. No.: CD008268. DOI: 10.1002/14651858.CD008268.pub2.

7) Guideline 117: Management of sore throat and indications for tonsillectomy. Edinburgh: Scottish Intercollegiate Guidelines Network; 2010 [cited 8 October 2014]. Available from: http://www.sign.ac.uk/pdf/sign117.pdf.

EPIGLOTTITIS AND SUPRAGLOTTITIS

Common Practice
Due to the serious nature of epiglottitis and supraglottitis, it is difficult to perform high-quality studies.
- Have a high index of clinical suspicion – see summary below.
- Patients in the community should be transferred to an appropriate emergency department urgently.
- Urgent specialist anaesthetic, ENT and, if applicable, paediatric opinions should be sought.
    - The ENT surgeon and anaesthetist will have to assess the airway, usually using a fibreoptic nasendoscope so airway equipment and personnel should be readied in anticipation.
- Patients should be assessed in a high-dependency area.
- Examination of the mouth and pharynx should not be undertaken by non-specialists as it may precipitate respiratory arrest, even in experienced hands.
- Administer humidified oxygen.
    - Nebulised adrenaline can be inhaled for those in respiratory distress.
- Intravenous broad-spectrum antibiotics should be administered as soon as possible.
    - One prospective randomised study of 55 paediatric patients[1] (before the introduction of *Haemophilus influenzae* vaccine) showed that a shorter course of ceftriaxone had good efficacy.
    - In one retrospective case series of 80 adult patients,[2] approximately 90% of patients received piperacillin or ticarcillin; the authors felt that these antibiotics were satisfactory.
- Intravenous steroid should be administered as soon as possible.
    - Some units will prescribe 8-10mg dexamethasone TDS for 24 to 48 hours, with dose tapering if needed.
- The patient should be kept nil by mouth.
- Admission to a critical care unit should be strongly considered.
- Consider elective intubation and prepare for the rare instances of emergency cricothyroidotomy or tracheostomy.[1,2]

NICE Guidelines
- None

EPIGLOTTITIS AND SUPRAGLOTTITIS

Summary
'Epiglottitis' is an acute infective condition of the epiglottis, which is part of the inlet of the larynx. 'Supraglottitis' is used to describe a more generalised inflammation of the entire inlet, including the arytenoid cartilages and other tissues.

Epiglottitis is predominantly seen in the paediatric population; in one study the age range was between 7 months and 6 years of age with a median age of 32 months.[1] Supraglottitis is typically seen in adult patients.

The main causative organism appears to be *Haemophilus influenzae* type B (Hib), but streptococcal species may also be responsible. The Hib vaccine has been given routinely in England since 1992 and has resulted in a reduction in cases of epiglottitis in the paediatric population.[2] Although it generally occurs in immunocompetent individuals, there are case reports of epiglottitis as a manifestation of haematological immune compromise *eg* leukaemia[5] or neutropenic sepsis. Some case reports suggest sporadic instances of epiglottitis due to atypical organisms such as *Staphyloccocus aureus*[6] and *Serratia marcescens*,[7] as well as tuberculous laryngitis in endemic areas.[8]

Our red flags for severe airway infection are:
1. Severe sore throat with aphagia or severe dysphagia (*ie* unable to swallow saliva)
2. Hoarse or no voice (*ie* hoarseness similar to shouting too much), often in the absence of stridor, which is a late sign

in a systemically unwell person who may have pyrexia, dehydration and other signs of sepsis. Any patient who has a severe sore throat where you cannot identify pharyngeal signs (tonsillitis, quinsy, trismus etc.) should be presumed to have epiglottitis until proven otherwise.

EPIGLOTTITIS AND SUPRAGLOTTITIS

References

1) Sawyer SM, Johnson PD, Hogg GG, Robertson CF, Oppedisano F, MacIness SJ, Gilbert GL. Successful treatment of epiglottitis with two doses of ceftriaxone. *Arch Dis Child*. 1994. 70(2): 129-32.

2) McVernon J, Slack MP, Ramsay ME. Changes in the epidemiology of epiglottitis following introduction of Haemophilus influenzae type b (Hib) conjugate vaccines in England: a comparison of two data sources. *Epidemiol Infect*. 2006.134(3):570-2.

3) Nakamura H, Tanaka H, Matsuda A, Fukushima E, Hasegawa M. Acute epiglottitis: a review of 80 patients. *J Laryngol Otol*. 2001 Jan;115(1):31-4.

4) Berger G, Landau T, Berger S, Finkelstein Y, Bernheim J, Ophir D. The rising incidence of adult acute epiglottitis and epiglottic abscess. *Am J Otolaryngol*. 2003 Nov-Dec;24(6):374-83.

5) Kagedan DJ, Haasz M, Kumar Chadha N, Vinod Mehta S. Epiglottitis as a presentation of leukemia in an adolescent. *Pediatr Emerg Care*. 2014. 30: 733-5.

6) Harris C, Sharkey L, Koshy G, Simler N, Karas JA. A rare case of epiglottitis due to Staphylococcus aureus in an adult. *Infect Dis Rep*. 2012. 4: e3.

7) Musham CK, Jarathi A, Agarwal A. Acute epiglottitis due to Serratia marcescens in an immunocompetent adult. *Am J Med Sci*. 2012. 344:153-4.

8) El Beltagi AH, Khera Ps, Alrabiah L, Al Shammari NF. Case report: acute tuberculous laryngitis presenting as acute epiglottitis. *Indian J Radiol Imaging*. 2011. 21: 284-6.

INFECTIOUS MONONUCLEOSIS (GLANDULAR FEVER)

Strongly Recommended
- Anti-herpes anti-virals should not be prescribed for infectious mononucleosis (IM).
    - One meta-analysis[1] (339 patients) showed that, although aciclovir appeared to inhibit oropharyngeal Epstein-Barr virus (EBV) replication, it did not affect symptom duration.[2]
- Regular steroids should not be prescribed for IM symptom control.
    - A Cochrane Review[3] that included seven trials found that, on 8/10 assessments of health improvement, there was no benefit derived from steroid.
    - Two of these trials found that steroid therapy reduced sore throat – but only transiently.

Suggested
- The diagnosis can be confirmed using agglutination tests or EBV-specific serological tests.[4]
    - Agglutination tests such as the Paul-Bunnell test have a variable sensitivity of between 50% for young children to 85% in adults.
    - EBV-specific serological tests vary in the exact method of analysis but sensitivity is higher.
    - Serological tests typically cost £6-8 whereas agglutination tests typically cost £4-5 in the NHS.

Common Practice
- It is common to advise patients to abstain from contact sports for three to six months. This relates to a risk of splenic rupture.[5]
- It is common to test liver function in cases of IM.
- Consider prescribing topical and systemic pain relief and fluids.

NICE Guidelines
- None

Summary
Infectious mononucleosis is an infective condition caused by the Epstein-Barr virus (EBV), a herpesvirus. It manifests as pharyngitis, fever, generalised lymphadenopathy, myalgia, headache and malaise. It is commonly seen in the adolescent-to-young adult age group and is transmitted in saliva. On the whole, symptoms are self-limiting. A small number of patients will go on to develop a rash, atypical lymphocytosis, splenomegaly and hepatomegaly with derangement of liver function. Admission may be required if there is poor oral intake. The illness lasts up to a few weeks but convalescence may be longer.

INFECTIOUS MONONUCLEOSIS (GLANDULAR FEVER)

References

1) Torre D, Tambini R. Acyclovir for treatment of infectious mononucleosis: a meta-analysis. *Scand J Infect Dis*. 1999; 31(6):543-7.

2) Tynell E, Aurelius E, Brandell A, Julander I, Wood M, Yao QY, Rickinson A, Akerlund B, Andersson J. Acyclovir and prednisolone treatment of acute infectious mononucleosis: a multicenter, double-blind, placebo-controlled study. *J Infect Dis*. 1996 Aug; 1 74(2):324-31.

3) Candy B, Hotopf M. Steroids for symptom control in infectious mononucleosis. *Cochrane Database Syst Rev*.
2006, Issue 3. Art. No.: CD004402. DOI: 10.1002/14651858.CD004402.pub2.

4) Hess RD. Routine Epstein-Barr virus diagnostics from the laboratory perspective: still challenging after 35 years. *J Clin Microbiol*. 2004; 42(8): 3381-87.

5) Rinderknecht AS, Pomerantz WJ. Spontaneous splenic rupture in infectious mononucleosis: case report and review of the literature. *Pediatr Emerg Care*. 2012. 28: 1377-9.

INGESTED FOREIGN BODY AND IMPACTED FOOD BOLUS

Common practice
Little high-quality evidence exists to guide management of this condition.
- Take a good history from the patient or family to ascertain symptoms suggestive of a foreign body, *eg* sudden onset while eating bony fish and unable to finish the meal, with regurgitation or drooling.
- Localisation of a foreign body by the patient does not always correlate well with its actual location.
    - Three studies[1-3] with a cumulative 538 patients conclude that patient localisation was more predictive if higher in the neck. One of these studies[1] reported a 97% positive predictive value (PPV) for sensations above the level of the cricoid cartilage. Lateralisation was also more accurate if higher in the neck (PPV 56-71%) and if the foreign body was found in a tonsil.[3]
- Perform a thorough examination of the oral cavity and oropharynx (as tolerated) including the tonsils and tongue base; perform nasendoscopy if indicated.
- Attempt removal of fish bones after application of local anaesthetic spray.
- Lateral soft-tissue neck radiographs should be taken only when indicated by clinical assessment, *eg* in a patient with persistent symptoms and an unremarkable examination
    - In patients with minor symptoms, imaging may not be indicated because of the high false positive rate. In two separate studies,[3, 4] both true positive and false positive rates were similar (approximately 30-35%).
    - Two studies[5, 6] report partially contradictory findings for the visibility of different types of fish bone on radiographs.
- There is no evidence to support the use of anti-spasmodic agents such as glucagon, Buscopan and diazepam in the treatment of impacted food bolus.[8-10]
- If foreign bodies have not dislodged spontaneously after 24 hours, or if patients have progressive symptoms, evaluation under general anaesthetic is warranted.
    - In some centres, soft food boluses will be managed with fibreoptic gastro-oesophagoscopy while hard foreign bodies will be managed with rigid oesophagoscopy.
    - Oesophageal foreign bodies that are unlikely to cause trauma, *ie* smaller smooth objects, may pass spontaneously.
- Button batteries must be removed from the throat urgently.
    - Effects vary from mild mucosal erosion to mucosal necrosis, rapid perforation and mediastinitis.

INGESTED FOREIGN BODY AND IMPACTED FOOD BOLUS

Summary

Foreign bodies 'stuck in the throat' are a common ENT referral occurring in all age groups. The range of foreign bodies encompasses soft foodstuffs, through to hard toys and coins in children and dentures in adults. According to one prospective study, the commonest sites for foreign bodies are (in order): the tonsil, upper third of the oesophagus, middle third of the oesophagus, hypopharynx, posterior third of the tongue, the vallecula, post-cricoid region and the posterior pharyngeal wall.[3] This did, however, change depending on the type of foreign body.

A further retrospective case review[7] found hypopharyngeal foreign bodies were more likely to occur in children under the age of 15. The majority of adults suffered impaction in the oesophagus. Impaction is thought to occur in cricopharyngeus due to muscle spasm. On the whole, most ENT surgeons will deal with proximal foreign bodies. Mid-to-distal oesophageal foreign bodies are generally referred to the general surgeons or gastroenterologists for management.

Patients, mainly adults and older children, may present with the complaint of swallowing a foreign body. In the younger age groups, this may be a witnessed event or only become apparent when symptoms develop. Common symptoms are dysphagia, regurgitation, odynophagia, and otalgia. Predisposing factors include neuromuscular incoordination, stricture formation and central nervous system disorders.

Foreign bodies may pass spontaneously. In one study, natural disimpaction of oesophageal foreign bodies occurred in 21% of patients.[7] Unfortunately, in a significant proportion of patients, rigid pharyngo-oesophagoscopy under general anaesthetic is required. If a diagnosis cannot be made at the time of initial rigid endoscopy, follow-up investigations (*eg* outpatient barium swallow or fibreoptic gastro-oesophagoscopy) should be arranged.

INGESTED FOREIGN BODY AND IMPACTED FOOD BOLUS

References

1) Yang CY and Yang CC. Subjective neck pain or foreign body sensation and the true location of foreign bodies in the pharynx. *Acta Otolaryngol*. 2014. [Epub ahead of print]. PMID: 25515966.

2) Connolly AA, Birchall M, Walsh-Waring GP, Moore-Gillon V. Ingested foreign bodies: patient-guided localization is a useful clinical tool. *Clin Otolaryngol Allied Sci*. 1992 Dec;17(6):520-4.

3) Jones NS, Lannigan FJ, Salama NY. Foreign bodies in the throat: a prospective study of 388 cases. *J Laryngol Otol*. 1991 Feb;105(2):104-8.

4) Marais J, Mitchell R, Wrightman AJ. The value of radiographic assessment for oropharyngeal foreign bodies. *J Laryngol Otol*. 1995 May;109(5):452-4.

5) Ell SR, Parker AJ. The radio-opacity of fish bones. *Clin Otolaryngol Allied Sci*. 1992 Dec;17(6):514-6.

6) Hone SW, Fenton J, Clarke E, Hamilton S, McShane D. The radio-opacity of fish bones: a cadaveric study. *Clin Otolaryngol Allied Sci*. 1995 Jun;20(3):234-5.

7) Tibbiing L, Stenquist M. Foreign bodies in the esophagus. A study of causative factors. *Dysphagia*. 1991;6(4):224-7.

8) Thomas L, Webb C, Duvvi S, Jones T, Reddy KT. Is buscopan effective in meat bolus obstruction? *Clin Otolaryngol*. 2005 Apr;30(2):183-5.

9) Mehta D, Attia M, Quintana E, Cronan K. Glucagon use for esophageal coin dislodgment in children: a prospective, double-blind, placebo— controlled trial. *Acad Emerg Med*. 2001 Feb;8(2): 200-3.

10) Tibbling L, Bjorkhoel A, Jansson E, Stenkvist M. Effect of spasmolytic drugs on esophageal foreign bodies. *Dysphagia*. 1995 Spring;10(2): 126-7.

NECK SPACE INFECTIONS

Common Practice
Little high-quality evidence exists for the management of these rare and life-threatening conditions.
- Patients in the community should be transferred to an appropriate emergency department urgently.
- Urgent specialist anaesthetic, ENT and, if applicable, paediatric opinions should be sought.
    - The ENT surgeon and anaesthetist will have to assess the airway, usually using a fibreoptic nasendoscope so airway equipment and personnel should be readied in anticipation.
- Patients should be assessed in a high-dependency area.
- Non-specialists should not undertake examination of the mouth and pharynx as it may precipitate respiratory arrest, even in experienced hands.
- Broad-spectrum intravenous antibiotics should be administered.
    - Two retrospective case series[1, 2] found that *Streptococcus viridans* was one of the commonest organisms cultured. Coagulase-negative *Staphylococcus*, *Klebsiella pneumoniae* and anaerobes were also cultured.
- Treatments to optimise the airway may help (steroids; nebulised adrenaline; humidified oxygen – see 'Epiglottitis').
- CT scanning with contrast is the investigation of choice.
    - A retrospective study[3] found that clinical evaluation alone under-estimated the extent of infection in 70% of patients.
    - Two retrospective analyses[4, 5] compared radiological findings with subsequent surgical findings. The CT false positive rate could be between 15-25%.

NICE Guidelines
- None.

NECK SPACE INFECTIONS

Summary

'Neck space infection' is a collective term for infections and abscesses affecting the potential compartments within the neck bound by muscles, mucosal and fascial layers and bony structures. They include prevertebral, retropharyngeal, parapharyngeal and submandibular (Ludwig's) abscesses. Peritonsillar abscess is also technically a neck space infection and is dealt with below.

Patients present with neck swelling, pain, dysphagia and odynophagia. There may be voice change and significant systemic upset. Examination may reveal neck swelling and erythema, soft palate oedema, medialisation of the tonsil and floor of mouth swelling, with potential for airway compromise. These infections arise from upper respiratory tract infection, tonsillopharyngitis, dental infections, retained foreign body and sometimes tuberculosis. In a minority of cases, no obvious cause is found.

If left untreated, neck space infections may lead to significant and life-threatening complications. Rupture into the pharynx with aspiration of contents, dissection into the mediastinum, airway obstruction and erosion into major blood vessels are all potential sequelae.

Management includes securing the airway in cases where it is compromised (elective intubation or emergency tracheostomy), intravenous antibiotics, intravenous steroids and drainage of pus.

NECK SPACE INFECTIONS

References

1) Boscolo-Rizzo P, Marchiori C, Montolli F, Vaglia A, Da Mosto MC. Deep Neck Infections: A Constant Challenge. *ORL J Otorhinolaryngol Relat Spec*. 2006 May 4;68(5):197-203.

2) Huang TT, Tseng FY, Yeh TH, Hsu CJ, Chen YS. Factors affecting the bacteriology of deep neck infection: a retrospective study of 128 patients. *Acta Otolaryngol*. 2006 Apr;126(4):396-401.

3) Crespo AN, Chone CT, Fonseca AS, Montenegro MC, Pereira R, Milani JA. Clinical versus computed tomography evaluation in the diagnosis and management of deep neck infection. *Sao Paulo Med J*. 2004 Nov 22(6): 259-63.

4) Smith JL 2nd, Hsu JM, Chang J. Predicting deep neck space abscess using computed tomography. *Am J Otolaryngol*. 2006 Jul-Aug;27(4):244-7.

5) Lazor JB, Cunningham MJ, Eavey RD, Weber AL. Comparison of computed tomography and surgical findings in deep neck infections. *Otolaryngol Head Neck Surg*. 1994 Dec;111(6):746-50.

PERITONSILLAR ABSCESS (QUINSY)

Suggested
- Peritonsillar abscesses should be drained soon after presentation
    - One study concluded that symptom resolution and recovery times were significantly shorter in those who undergo surgical drainage of their peritonsillar abscess.[1, 2]
- Incision and drainage may lead to quicker resolution of symptoms but it may be more difficult for non-specialists to become confident in using this technique.
    - One prospective study of 75 patients[3] found that 92% of those undergoing incision and drainage could drink water two hours after the procedure, compared with 8% in the aspiration group and none in the intravenous antibiotic group.
- Around 10% of patients will require further drainage, regardless of drainage technique.[4, 5]
- A combination of local anaesthetic infiltration and topical spray may provide better anaesthesia than topical spray alone.
    - A small trial of 30 patients[6] demonstrated significantly lower mean pain scores for patients receiving both infiltration and spray, compared to those receiving spray alone (in both drainage techniques).
- Consider a single dose of corticosteroid as an adjunct to antibiotic therapy and drainage.
    - One review[7] analysed two small randomised, placebo-controlled trials and one larger retrospective cohort study. On various measures such as inter-incisor distance, return to normal diet and length of stay, a single dose of IV steroid transiently improved symptoms. There was also a small decrease in the length of stay. (The trials used 2-3mg/kg methylprednisolone and 10mg dexamethasone.)
- Consider treatment with penicillin and metronidazole if not contra-indicated (follow your local policy).
    - A few studies[8-10] have examined the microbiological findings from culture of aspirated pus. The single largest study[10] of 577 cases found that *Streptococci* were isolated in about half of all cultures, with anaerobes in about one quarter.
- Intra-oral ultrasound may help to diagnose peritonsillar abscess but due to the need for specialist equipment and personnel, this has not gained popularity in the UK.[11, 12]

PERITONSILLAR ABSCESS (QUINSY)

NICE Guidelines
- None.

Summary
Peritonsillar abscess (also known as 'quinsy') is a painful condition where infection tracks into the space between the fibrous capsule of the upper pole of the tonsil and the superior constrictor muscle of the pharynx. It may represent the midpoint of a spectrum of disease from tonsillopharyngitis to parapharyngeal abscess. Drainage and antibiotic therapy are the mainstay of management because they improve time to recovery and avoid progression to a severe, airway-threatening infection.

Our red flags for severe airway infection are:
1. Severe sore throat with aphagia or severe dysphagia (*ie* unable to swallow saliva)
2. Hoarse or no voice (*ie* hoarseness similar to shouting too much), often in the absence of stridor, which is a late sign

in a systemically unwell person who may have pyrexia, dehydration and other signs of sepsis. Any patient who has a severe sore throat where you cannot identify pharyngeal signs (tonsillitis, quinsy, trismus etc.) should be presumed to have epiglottitis until proven otherwise.

PERITONSILLAR ABSCESS (QUINSY)

References

1) Powell J and Wilson JA. An evidence-based review of peritonsillar abscess. *Clin Otolaryngol*. 2012. 37: 136-145.

2) Tachibana T, Orita Y, Abe-Fujisawa I, Ogawara Y, Matsuyama Y, Shimizu A, Nakada M, Sato Y, Nishizaki K. Prognostic factors and effect of early surgical drainage in patients with peritonsillar abscess. *J Infect Chemother*. 2014. 20:722-5.

3) Nwe TT, Singh B. Management of pain in peritonsillar abscess. *J Laryngol Otol*. 2000 Oct;114(10):765-7.

4) Stringer SP, Shaefer SD, Close LG. A randomized trial for outpatient management of peritonsillar abscess. *Arch Otolaryngol Head Neck Surg*. 114: 296-298.

5) Herzon FS. Harris P Mosher Award Thesis. Peritonsillar abscess: incidence, current management practices, and a proposal for treatment guidelines. *Laryngoscope*. 1995 Aug;105(8 Pt 3 Suppl 74):1-17.

6) Tandon S, Roe J, Lancaster J. A randomized trial of local anaesthetic in treatment of quinsy. *Clin Otolaryngol Allied Sci*. 2004 Oct;29(5):535-7.

7) Hardman JC, McCulloch NA, Nankivell P. Do corticosteroids improve outcome in peritonsillar abscess? *Laryngoscope*. 2014 Sep doi: 10.1002/lary.24936 [Epub ahead of print].

8) Maharaj D, Rajah V, Hemsley S. Management of peritonsillar abscess. *J Laryngol Otol*. 1991 Sep;105(9):743-5.

9) Prior A, Montgomery P, Mitchelmore I, Tabaqchali S. The microbiology and antibiotic treatment of peritonsillar abscesses. *Clin Otolaryng Aliied Sci*. 1995 Jun;20(3):219-23.

10) Repanos C, Mukherjee P, Alwahab Y. Role of microbiological studies in management of peritonsillar abscess. *J Laryngol Otol*. 2009. 123: 877-9.

11) Scott PMJ, Loftus WK, Kew J, Ahuja A, Yue V, van Hasselt CA. Diagnosis of peritonsillar infections: a prospective study of ultrasound, computerized tomography and clinical diagnosis. *J Laryngol Otol*. 1999. 113: 229-32.

12) Araujo Filho BC, Sakae FA, Sennes LU, Imamura R, de Menezes MR. Intraoral and transcutaneous cervical ultrasound in the differential diagnosis of peritonsillar cellulitis and abscesses. *Rev Bras Otorhinolaryngol*. 2006. 72:377-81.

POSTOPERATIVE CARE

POSTOPERATIVE CARE INTRODUCTION

This section outlines some common ENT procedures and gives details of the patient's likely postoperative course. It describes the most common complications that occur early in the postoperative period, and gives brief information about their management.

Please note that it is not a complete guide to the operative procedures or their complications, and individual surgeons' practice may vary.

Always check the surgeon's operation note, whether you are discharging a patient or a patient has re-presented with a possible complication.

Consent for an operation should only be taken by a surgeon able to perform the procedure, or someone specially trained to do so.

OTOLOGY

GROMMET INSERTION

Summary
Grommets are small plastic rings or tubes. They are inserted into the tympanic membrane to ventilate the middle ear. The most common kind used are Shah grommets; T-tube grommets offer longer-term ventilation. A small incision (myringotomy) is made in the antero-inferior quadrant of the tympanic membrane, and a grommet is inserted.

Indication
Presence of glue ear causing persistent conductive hearing loss (see NICE Clinical Guideline CG60). Glue ear is also known as otitis media with effusion (OME) or secretory otitis media.

Anaesthetic
General; may be performed under local in cooperative adults.

Post-op stay
Day-case.

Postoperative care and common early complications
Pain – minimal.

Bleeding – minimal, self-limiting.

Water precautions – cotton-wool and Vaseline ear plugs for showering or bathing. No swimming for 4 weeks, subsequently ear plugs or head band/cap should be used.

Post op infection – manifests as otorrhoea, usually without pain. This should be treated with ear drops (not oral antibiotics). Ciprofloxacin drops are usually preferred, although the risk of ototoxicity is minimal.

Postoperative medications
Simple analgesia. Ear drops are occasionally prescribed.

Follow up
Routine postoperative review, with an audiogram on arrival.

MYRINGOPLASTY

Summary
Repair of a tympanic membrane perforation to prevent infections. The middle ear is approached down the ear canal (permeatal), or using a postauricular or endaural incision to widen access. The tympanic membrane is raised up, and a graft, usually of temporal fascia or tragal perichondrium, is inserted under the edges of the perforation and acts as a scaffold for healing.

Indication
Mucosal chronic otitis media – a discharging tympanic membrane perforation.

Anaesthetic
General, very occasionally under local.

Post-op stay
Day-case or one-night stay.

Postoperative care and common early complications
Pain – minimal.

Removal of sutures – 5 to 7 days. If non-absorbable sutures are used in an endaural or postauricular approach.

Removal of packs – a ribbon soaked in BIPP (bismuth iodoform paraffin paste) or ointment is usually left in the ear canal. This is removed at around 2 weeks in clinic.

Bleeding – usually minimal; some oozing may occur from incision.

Head bandage – may be used if an external incision is made. Usually removed the following day.

Water precautions – cotton-wool and Vaseline ear plugs for showering or bathing. No swimming until clinical review.

MYRINGOPLASTY

Postoperative care and common early complications (continued)

Otorrhoea – coloured discharge may be due to packing, if BIPP is used. Subsequent infection should be treated promptly with drops, as it may lead to graft failure. Avoid removing BIPP packing out-of-hours: discuss during working hours with the operating surgeon or the on-call registrar. Mild cases of discharge may not warrant removal of BIPP packing, which is placed in the ear to support the graft.

Dizziness/tinnitus – mild, usually transient.

Postoperative medications
Simple analgesia.

Follow up
Patients are usually seen 2 weeks post-operatively in clinic for pack removal.

MASTOIDECTOMY

Summary
The mastoid bone is drilled out and the middle ear is explored, to eradicate disease (cholesteatoma or chronically inflamed mucosa). The posterior ear canal wall may be left intact, or removed, resulting in an "open cavity".

Indication
Treatment of chronic otitis media, with or without cholesteatoma.

Anaesthetic
General.

Post-op stay
One-night stay.

Postoperative care and common early complications
Pain – mild.

Removal of sutures – 5 to 7 days if non-absorbable sutures have been used. Incision may be in front (endaural) or behind the ear (postauricular).

Removal of packs – ear canal packing is usually removed in clinic around 2 weeks post-operatively. If part of the packing falls out prior to the clinic appointment, advice is to trim the loose end and leave the rest in place.

Bleeding – minimal and self-limiting.

Head bandage – if used, removed the next morning.

Water precautions – Vaseline and cotton-wool in conchal bowl during bathing or showering.

Otorrhoea – mild, may be due to the ear pack if BIPP has been used.

Dizziness – mild, usually transient.

MASTOIDECTOMY

Postoperative care and common early complications (continued)
Taste disturbance – due to injury to the chorda tympani. Results in a metallic taste which frequently improves over time.

Facial weakness – rare. May be due to several causes. Contact the operating surgeon for guidance.

Postoperative medications
Simple analgesia.

Follow up
Patients are usually seen 2 weeks post-operatively for pack removal.

STAPEDECTOMY

Summary
Surgical treatment to treat conductive hearing loss due to otosclerosis, which leads to fixation of the stapes footplate. The stapes superstructure is removed and a hole (fenestration) is made in the footplate, using a drill or laser. A piston is placed into the fenestration and fixed to the long process of the incus.

Indication
Otosclerosis leading to significant conductive hearing loss.

Anaesthetic
General, or local with sedation.

Post-op stay
One-night stay.

Postoperative care and common early complications
Pain – mild.

Removal of sutures – only if permeatal approach is not used

Removal of packs – ear canal packing is usually removed in clinic around 2 weeks post-operatively. If part of the packing falls out prior to the clinic appointment, advice is to trim the loose end and leave the rest in place.

Bleeding – minimal and self-limiting.

Head bandage – if used, removed the next morning.

Dizziness – mild, usually transient.

Taste disturbance – uncommon; due to injury to the chorda tympani. Results in a metallic taste which frequently improves over time.

Facial weakness – very rare.

Postoperative medications
Simple analgesia.

Follow up
Patients are usually seen 2 weeks post-operatively for pack removal.

RHINOLOGY

SEPTOPLASTY

Summary
Procedure to straighten the cartilage and bone of the nasal septum. A flap of mucoperichondrium is raised to expose the septal cartilage, which is mobilised and/or selectively resected to alter its shape.

Indication
Unilateral nasal blockage, as part of a rhinoplasty procedure, or occasionally for access in endoscopic nasal surgery.

Anaesthetic
General.

Post-op stay
Day-case.

Postoperative care and common early complications
Pain – mild

Nasal blockage – may last for around 2 weeks.

Bleeding – usually minimal and self-limiting. Blood-stained discharge for up to 2 weeks after the procedure is expected. Significant bleeding may be due to turbinate injury.

Removal of packs – nasal packs (if used) are removed a few hours postoperatively, or the following morning.

Splints – usually made of silicone material. If inserted, remove 1 week after surgery. Kept in place with a through-and-through suture – requires cutting prior to removal. If no splints are placed, absorbable sutures are normally used.

Nose blowing – avoid for 1 week post-operatively; sneeze through mouth

Postoperative medications
Simple analgesia. Some surgeons prescribe nasal douching.

Follow up
Routine outpatient review.

SEPTORHINOPLASTY

Summary
Procedure to alter the external nasal appearance, improve nasal airway, or both. Can be performed via an open or an endonasal approach, depending on the severity of deformity and the surgeon's preference. The septum is straightened (see above) and the nasal bones may be fractured by osteotomies to allow correction of deformities. The alar cartilages can be resected and/or sutured to change the shape of the nasal tip.

Indication
Aesthetic improvement and/or to improve nasal blockage (congenital or acquired through trauma).

Anaesthetic
General.

Post-op stay
Day-case or one-night stay.

Postoperative care and common early complications
Pain – usually mild, however recovery can be quite uncomfortable due to congestion and swelling.

Bleeding – usually minimal and self-limiting. Blood stained discharge up to 2 weeks after procedure is expected. Significant bleeding may be due to turbinate injury.

Nasal blockage – may last for around 2 weeks, or longer in extensive procedures.

Removal of sutures – Sutures in the nasal cavity will dissolve. If an open-approach procedure is performed, the columellar incision is usually closed with 6/0 nylon or prolene, removed at around 5-7 days.

External splint – removed in outpatient clinic in 1 week.

Removal of packs – nasal packs (if used) are removed the day after surgery.

Splints – If inserted, are removed 1 week after surgery. Kept in place with through-and-through suture – requires cutting prior to removal.

SEPTORHINOPLASTY

Postoperative care and common early complications (continued)
Bruising – periorbital and facial bruising and swelling is common, and settles after 10 to 14 days.

Nose blowing – avoid for 1 week post-operatively; sneeze through mouth.

Postoperative medications
Simple analgesia. Some surgeons prescribe nasal douching.

Follow up
Around 7 days in clinic for splint or suture removal.

FUNCTIONAL ENDOSCOPIC SINUS SURGERY (FESS)

Summary
Endoscopic surgery allows the removal of nasal polyps and the exploration and opening of the paranasal sinuses to improve their drainage or resect diseased tissue.

Indication
Chronic rhinosinusitis with or without nasal polyposis, which has not responded to maximal medical therapy. FESS may also be performed for tumour resection, or access to the skull base and beyond.

Anaesthetic
General.

Post-op stay
Day-case or one-night stay.

Postoperative care and common early complications
Pain – mild. The patient will experience congestion for some weeks postoperatively.

Removal of sutures – nil; no external scars, bruising or swelling.

Removal of packs – nasal packs (if used) are removed the day after surgery.

Bleeding – usually minimal and self-limiting. Blood-stained discharge for up to 2 weeks after procedure is expected.

Nose blowing – avoid for 1 week post-operatively; sneeze through mouth.

Postoperative medications
Simple analgesia. Usually steroid nasal drops or spray is prescribed, with or without nasal douching, as a long-term medication. Occasionally antibiotics or oral steroids are prescribed.

Follow up
Routine outpatient review.

HEAD AND NECK SURGERY

TONSILLECTOMY

Summary
Removal of the palatine tonsils, with steel or electrosurgical instruments. May be performed in conjunction with adenoidectomy (see below).

Indication
Recurrent acute tonsillitis (see SIGN Guideline 117), quinsy, obstructive sleep apnoea, or under suspicion of malignancy.

Anaesthetic
General.

Post-op stay
Usually day-case.

Postoperative care and common early complications
Pain – severe, lasting up to 2 weeks. Regular analgesia is essential to allow a normal diet. May worsen on days 2-3 post-op. May include referred otalgia.

Removal of sutures – nil; silk ties may be used for haemostasis but are not removed.

Bleeding – reactionary bleeding is rare, but mandates return to theatre. Secondary bleeding occurs in around 4% of cases, roughly 7 days postoperatively. Patients must be told to attend the hospital immediately, and are kept in for observation. Persistent bleeding is an indication to take the patient to theatre for haemostasis.

Eating and drinking – as soon as tolerated. Patients should be advised to maintain a normal diet.

Appearance – the back of the throat will appear white or yellow. This is normal and is not a sign of infection.

TONSILLECTOMY

Postoperative medications
Analgesia: paracetamol 1g qds, ibuprofen 400mg tds, codeine phosphate 30-60 mg qds +/- bendyzamine throat spray, in adults. *Codeine must NOT be prescribed to patients under 18 years old.*

Follow up
Nil, unless for histology, or occasionally for obstructive sleep apnoea.

ADENOIDECTOMY

Summary
Removal of adenoid tissue from the postnasal space (usually in children). This can be performed with an adenoid curette or with an electrosurgical technique such as suction diathermy. Often performed in conjunction with tonsillectomy (see previous).

Indication
Obstructive sleep apnoea in children (in combination with tonsillectomy), in conjunction with ventilation tube insertion, or occasionally for nasal blockage.

Anaesthetic
General.

Post-op stay
One-night stay if for OSA.

Postoperative care and common early complications
Pain – mild.

Bleeding – rare, but patients should be advised to attend hospital urgently if this occurs.

Nasal regurgitation of fluids when drinking – may occur due to widening of the velopharyngeal sphincter. This generally resolves spontaneously.

Postoperative medications
Simple analgesia only.

Follow up
Nil – unless for ventilation tube follow-up (see previous).

RIGID (PAN-) ENDOSCOPY

Summary
Endoscopic examination of the larynx, pharynx and/or oesophagus, using rigid metal tubular scopes.

Indication
For visualisation of the larynx, pharynx and oesophagus, biopsy for suspected malignancy, removal of foreign bodies, or laryngeal microsurgery and laser surgery.

Anaesthetic
General.

Post-op stay
Day-case, or occasionally one-night stay in frail patients / complex cases.

Postoperative care and common early complications
Pain – mild. The patient may experience sore gums / teeth, neck stiffness or mild sore throat for up to 7 days.

Bleeding – a small amount if biopsies are taken.

Eating and drinking – the patient may be kept nil by mouth immediately afterwards, followed by gradual reintroduction of oral intake. Check the operation note. If perforation is suspected, the patient may be kept nil by mouth and fed via a nasogastric (NG) tube for a more extended period.

Perforation – patients with postoperative chest pain, back pain, tachycardia, dysphagia or surgical emphysema may have sustained a perforation. The patient should be fed via NG only and started on IV antibiotics. This is a potentially life-threatening complication.

Voice – absolute voice rest is advised for 24-48 hours after vocal cord biopsy, followed by relative voice rest (minimal talking, no whispering or shouting) for a week.

Postoperative medications
Simple analgesia only.

Follow up
Dependent on indication – 2 weeks if a biopsy is taken.

THYROIDECTOMY AND HEMITHYROIDECTOMY

Summary
Removal of one or both lobes of the thyroid gland. A horizontal skin-crease incision is made in the neck and the strap muscles are divided. The thyroid gland is dissected out, identifying and preserving the recurrent laryngeal nerve which runs posteriorly.

Indication
Suspected or confirmed thyroid malignancy, Graves' disease not responsive to medical treatment, or large benign goitre leading to compression or cosmetic concern.

Anaesthetic
General.

Post-op stay
Usually a one-night stay, occasionally two nights.

Postoperative care and common early complications
Pain – mild to moderate.

Removal of sutures – absorbable or non-absorbable sutures may be used. If needed, sutures are removed 7 days postoperatively.

Bleeding – bleeding into the operative site is uncommon, but can lead to haematoma and airway obstruction due to laryngeal oedema. Suture removal equipment must be available at the bedside. If haematoma with airway compromise occurs, get senior anaesthetic support, sit the patient upright, deliver high-flow oxygen, and open and evacuate the neck at the bedside. The patient should be intubated and returned to theatre for haemostasis.

Recurrent laryngeal nerve injury – may lead to hoarseness. This may be temporary due to neurapraxia, or more rarely permanent due to transection of the nerve.

THYROIDECTOMY AND HEMITHYROIDECTOMY

Postoperative care and common early complications (continued)
Hypocalcaemia – due to removal of, or damage to parathyroid glands. Postoperative hypocalcaemia is more common after total thyroidectomy, and calcium is therefore measured at least once postoperatively. Check local protocols. Hypocalcaemic patients, particularly if symptomatic, may require IV calcium gluconate infusion with cardiac monitoring.

Postoperative medications
Analgesia: paracetamol 1g qds, ibuprofen 400mg tds, with or without codeine. Oral calcium +/- vitamin D may be prescribed if needed. In total thyroidectomy, the patient is started on levothyroxine (liothyronine (T3) if malignancy).

Follow up
Review in clinic in 2 weeks for histology.

SUPERFICIAL PAROTIDECTOMY

Summary
Removal of benign parotid tumours, with a cuff of normal tissue. The parotid gland is exposed and the facial nerve is identified at its exit from the stylomastoid foramen. The nerve is followed meticulously as it runs through the gland, and the tissue superficial to the nerve is resected.

Indication
Benign parotid tumours such as pleomorphic adenoma.

Anaesthetic
General.

Post-op stay
Usually a one-night stay, occasionally two nights.

Postoperative care and common early complications
Pain – mild to moderate.

Drain – monitor output closely and refer to the operation note for when this should be removed.

Removal of sutures – absorbable or non-absorbable sutures may be used. If needed, sutures are removed 5-7 days postoperatively.

Bleeding – high drain output or haematoma may necessitate return to theatre for haemostasis.

Salivary collection – can usually be managed conservatively.

Facial nerve injury – may be temporary, due to traction on the nerve, or permanent if the nerve is divided. Paralysis may be partial if only a branch has been damaged. Read the operation note and contact the operating surgeon.

Numbness of inferior pinna – quite common, as the greater auricular nerve may have to be divided for access.

Postoperative medications
Analgesia: paracetamol 1g qds, ibuprofen 400mg tds, with or without codeine.

Follow up
Review in clinic in 2 weeks for histology.

SUBMANDIBULAR GLAND EXCISION

Summary
Removal of the submandibular gland. A skin-crease incision is made two finger-breadths below the mandible. The incision is deepened to the capsule of the gland, and the dissection continues close to the gland.

Indication
Benign or malignant tumours (may be performed as part of a more extensive neck dissection). Also performed for recurrent submandibular gland infection or obstruction by stones.

Anaesthetic
General.

Post-op stay
Usually a one-night stay.

Postoperative care and common early complications
Pain – mild to moderate.

Drain – monitor output and refer to the operation note for when this should be removed.

Removal of sutures – absorbable or non-absorbable sutures may be used. If needed, sutures are removed 5-7 days postoperatively.

Bleeding – high drain output or haematoma may necessitate return to theatre for haemostasis.

Marginal mandibular nerve injury – leads to weakness of the corner of the mouth. This is quite often temporary but can be permanent.

Other nerve injury – may lead to tongue weakness or numbness (both are rare).

Postoperative medications
Analgesia: paracetamol 1g qds, ibuprofen 400mg tds, with or without codeine.

Follow up
Review in clinic in 2 weeks for histology.

STAPLING OF PHARYNGEAL POUCH

Summary
Opening of a pharyngeal pouch into the oesophagus to treat its symptoms. The pouch neck is visualised using a diverticuloscope, and a stapler is used to divide the wall between the pouch and the upper oesophagus.

Indication
Pharyngeal pouch leading to regurgitation, aspiration or other symptoms. Most patients are elderly.

Anaesthetic
General.

Post-op stay
Usually a one-night stay.

Postoperative care and common early complications
Pain – mild to moderate sore throat.

Perforation – may occur due to trauma from the scope or failure of the staple line. The patient may have a nasogastric tube inserted intraoperatively in case it is required for feeding. See above under *Rigid endoscopy*.

Diet – the patient is often kept nil-by-mouth overnight, followed by water and then soft diet. Check the operation note.

Postoperative medications
Analgesia.

Follow up
Routine outpatient review.

TRACHEOSTOMY

Summary
Creation of a surgical airway into the trachea. A horizontal incision is made in the neck and the strap muscles are divided in the midline. The thyroid isthmus is retracted or divided. A window is cut into the trachea and a suitable tracheostomy tube is inserted.

Indication
Long-term ventilation – to reduce dead space, prevent subglottic stenosis and allow bronchial toilet. To allow weaning from ventilation. Airway obstruction (the procedure differs in emergency tracheostomy).

Anaesthetic
General except in acute airway obstruction.

Post-op stay
One-night stay (although most patients require ongoing hospital care).

Postoperative care and common early complications
Care of the tracheostomised patient requires significant training and is covered only in brief.

Bleeding – may be mild, around the wound, or due to granulation tissue in the trachea, but rarely there can be serious delayed bleeding due to vascular erosion.

Infection – quite common: the tracheostomy site requires diligent nursing care.

Airway obstruction – blockage of the tube with secretions is the most common cause. *In the event of tube obstruction, call for senior and anaesthetic help.* Remove the inner cannula, which should open the airway. If this is unsuccessful, deflate the cuff (the patient may be able to breathe via the normal route unless the tracheostomy was performed for airway obstruction).

Dislodgement – in the first few days after tracheostomy, this can be catastrophic, as the tract is not well-developed. *In the event of dislodgement, call for senior and anaesthetic help.* Lie the patient flat with their neck extended. Try to insert a spare tube using tracheal dilators +/- a gum elastic bougie.

General care – the patient MUST be cared for by nurses experienced in tracheostomy care. The tracheostomy tube inserted initially should have an inner cannula, and be suctioned regularly. The patient should have humidified oxygen with intermittent nebulised saline. This is to prevent mucus plug occlusion, which is a particular problem in the initial period.

Printed in Great Britain
by Amazon